UNDERSTANDING AND LIVING WITH BRAIN DAMAGE

UNDERSTANDING AND LIVING WITH BRAIN DAMAGE

By

PATRICK E. LOGUE, Ph.D.

Assistant Professor of Psychology
Duke University Medical Center
Durham, North Carolina

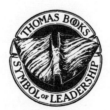

CHARLES C THOMAS • PUBLISHER
Springfield • *Illinois* • *U.S.A.*

Published and Distributed Throughout the World by
CHARLES C THOMAS • PUBLISHER
Bannerstone House
301-327 East Lawrence Avenue, Springfield, Illinois, U.S.A.

© *1975, by* CHARLES C THOMAS • PUBLISHER
ISBN 0-398-03419-2 (cloth)
ISBN 0-398-03420-6 (paper)
Library of Congress Catalog Card Number: 74-34256

With THOMAS BOOKS *careful attention is given to all details of manufacturing and design. It is the Publisher's desire to present books that are satisfactory as to their physical qualities and artistic possibilities and appropriate for their particular use.* THOMAS BOOKS *will be true to those laws of quality that assure a good name and good will.*

Printed in the United States of America
R-1

Library of Congress Cataloging in Publication Data
Logue, Patrick E
   Understanding and living with brain damage.

   Includes index.
   1. Brain damage.   I. Title. [DNLM: 1. Brain
damage, Chronic--Popular works. WL340 L832u]
RC386.2.L64   616.8   74-34256
ISBN 0-398-03419-2
ISBN 0-398-03420-6 pbk.

PREFACE

BRAIN DAMAGE AND HUMAN BEHAVIOR

Human behavior is a complex and little understood process. Although in a self-conscious way, people have always felt that "the proper study of mankind is man himself," much of what we do remains confusing even to ourselves.

Although there is room for argument even here, most would agree that man is unique in his ability to think and to reason. The reasoning process is centered in the grey, spongy mass of cerebral tissue of the brain. When accident, disease, or birth injury damages the brain, the person's behavior and life can be altered, sometimes beyond recognition.

The term *brain damage* or organicity conveys very little psychologically or medically. Unfortunately the emotions aroused by the words are profound to the listener. The parent, teacher, or spouse who is told that one close to them is brain damaged is usually afraid and somehow feels that the patient is doomed to an unproductive and wasted existence. But the term brain damage is vague and threatening. Brain damage is not one condition with a uniform and depressing set of symptoms. The consequences of brain damage vary greatly and depend on many factors. The nature of the illness, the age of the individual, and the area of the brain injured all influence the effects and the prognosis. The behavioral changes for the individual may run the gamut from profound to barely detectable with the most precise medical or psychological instruments.

The diagnosis and treatment of neurological conditions are, of course, medical. The emotional, reasoning, and behavioral effects and limitations that present themselves once the patient has been seen and treated by a physician must also be dealt with. This book is an attempt to explain in easily understood terms the practical effects of neurological conditions on the individual and on his family, and to assist, if possible, in the adjustment. Damage to the brain, if only as part of the natural aging process, is part of everyone's experience.

The chapter headings will correspond to some of the more common neurological conditions in adults and children. The same basic format will be followed in each chapter. First, the condition will be described in easily understood terms. Second, the possible behavioral consequences of the condition will be discussed with emphasis on their practical relevance to the individual, personally and vocationally. It is the strong belief of the writer that the significance of a behavioral limitation depends not only on its presence or absence but more importantly on the conditions under which the person works and lives. For example, a minor difficulty in coordinating the left and right hands may be of no consequence to a teacher but may be disastrous to a professional ball player. Suggestions will be made as to management and programming possibilities within the home. Finally, possible sources of professional help and treatment will be discussed. Where helpful, a complete psychological report illustrating the condition is included. Since certain symptoms are common to many disorders, one general chapter on common effects of brain damage is provided. This chapter should be read, regardless of the problem of interest. The contents page of the book is designed as a checklist for the physician. Where a special condition or category is characteristic of a patient, the chapters which deal with those conditions can be marked. After Chapter 1 and the chapters suggested by your physician have been read, the final chapter can help clarify or re-emphasize the important parts of those chapters.

CONTENTS

(Physician May Check Those Chapters
Relevant to Specific Problem)

UNDERSTANDING
AND LIVING WITH
BRAIN DAMAGE

GENERAL EFFECTS OF
DAMAGE TO THE BRAIN

THIS chapter deals with the general effects of damage to the brain. It is designed as an introduction to any of the chapters on specific conditions. It is divided into several sections:

1. Left Hemisphere Effects
2. Right Hemisphere Effects
3. Adaptive Functioning
4. Memory Effects
5. Other Treatment Possibilities
6. Emotional/Therapeutic Support
7. Sources of Help

BEHAVIORAL EFFECTS

The brain is divided into left and right sides. Each side controls the opposite side of the body and involves different thinking processes. Let us examine objectively, if possible, the significant effects of damage to each side.

Left Hemisphere Effects

The left side of the brain has often been called the *dominant* or *major* hemisphere. Not only does the left hemisphere control the right side and hand, usually the preferred side, but it nearly always is the controlling mechanism for the understanding and expression of language, written and spoken. Damage to the left hemisphere, then, typically causes some change in the ability to use, remember, and retrieve language. Disruption of language abilities from damage to the brain is called *aphasia*. Because of the importance of language in the child and in the adult in our culture, interruption of the delicate process that it represents can

3

only be described as catastrophic. Consider how it would be to awaken in the morning changed from a fully functioning, middle-aged adult to someone trapped in your own body, unable perhaps to utter an intelligible sound or even to understand the words written or spoken to you. The absence of physical pain associated with the loss of speech makes the loss of speech and functions more disturbing. Not all aphasias are so profound and often the recovery potential with proper speech therapy is excellent, but the feeling of tremendous loss and frustration must always be present at first. Even minor difficulty in finding the right word can cause frustration, depression, and anger.

Because aphasia can occur in many organic conditions which influence the left hemisphere, it is handled at length in Chapter 4.

Along with language functions, some studies have found that the left hemisphere is critical in the carrying out of sequences or chains of activities. Such skills are necessary where a task involves more than one step or when each step must follow another in a predetermined order or time. Many human activities, even as simple as washing dishes or writing a letter, do involve such a fixed chain of actions. For example, in writing a letter the person might

1. find the paper and pen
2. sit down at an appropriate place
3. address the top of the letter
4. structure the letter in some reasonable way
5. address the envelope and put a stamp on it
6. mail the letter.

Disruption of this ability may leave the person unable to preplan and to carry out that plan in a logical sequence. He may do the first steps of sequence and then be unable to go on. For example, if the individual is fixing a car, he may take out the jack, especially if it is an old familiar action, but may be unable to go further in the necessary chain of activities. He may then remain immobilized and frustrated.

Right Hemisphere — Spacial, Sensory, Motor Effects

The effects of damage to the right side of the brain usually disrupt spacial functioning. The patient is often unable to deal effectively with two- or three-dimensional space. For example, the ability to draw, copy, and remember forms or to construct objects is often profoundly effected. The patient may become lost easily. He may lose his car in the parking lot. A draftsman may be unable to understand even a simple blueprint. Speech, once the acute phase of the illness is over, may be relatively uneffected. Intelligence test scores may show little effect. Inability to effectively use the left side (arm or leg) can occur. Sensations of touch and pain may be so influenced that the patient can severely injure his hand without realizing it. The same would be true, of course, in left hemisphere damage.

To some extent, also, musical perception and spacial memory, ie.e memory for faces, may be influenced by right hemisphere damage. Creative and intuitive reasoning have been suggested as being right hemisphere functions, but the evidence is slight at present.

Adaptive Functioning Loss (Right and Left Hemisphere)

It would appear that the individual who suffers damage to the right hemisphere is relatively lucky, since speech loss is critical. Most medical workers act on that premise. But the relatively intact speech and intelligence test (IQ) scores of the patient within the circumscribed confines of the hospital may mask a more subtle deficit (the loss of adaptive abilities) which only become apparent as more demands and less structure are placed on the patient.

Speech, in typical social interaction, complex as it is, is old learned behavior. Most of our daily talking is simply a replay of words and automatic phrases used many times before. When we ask someone "How are you?" we are certainly not communicating much beyond a polite acknowledgement of their presence; we would probably be somewhat offended if they really told us, "how they are." Few demands are placed on the individual to solve problems or to deal quickly and alertly with his environment. The hospital environment is deliberately structured in such a fashion as to remove most elements of

ambiguity or choice. The patient choices are limited to whether to
have breakfast at 6 AM or to argue with the nurse. Patients who
attempt to make too many of their own decisions are not favorably
thought of. Similarly, IQ scores typically represent old stored
knowledge, i.e. what is the color of an apple? Intelligence test
scores may seem to convey more than they really do and like most
complex tasks, can be influenced positively and negatively by
many variables. The individual who retains his verbal skills can,
within a structured context, seem more alert and able than he is.
However, if the individual is placed in a life situation in which he
must "think on his feet" and respond to a new or emergency
situation, a very different kind of ability is brought into play. The
stroke patient with a verbal IQ of 100 could be totally
psychologically immobilized if a kitchen fire starts.

It has been found that in severe organic conditions, the problem
solving or adaptive abilities are sharply curtailed. If the home or
job requires precise analysis, rapid shifting, and decision making,
the patient can become completely frustrated and upset. Such a
catastrophic reaction is sometimes alarming and unexpected,
since the patient, in ordinary conversation, seems relatively
unchanged and quite capable.

Vocational Implication of Adaptive Loss

Although any life situation requires problem solving to some
extent, the frequency, difficulty, and consequences of those
decision vary enormously. None of us would prefer to have the
services of a pilot, therapist, or physician whose ability to make
rapid, precise, accurate responses to the needs of those dependent
on his skills were impaired to the slightest degree. Such
individuals are constantly responsible for the well-being of many
others on a daily basis. Jobs and life situations that are more
stereotyped and routine in their personal demands on the patient
may be far more suitable and even highly therapeutic within the
medical and physical limitations that remain. Less demanding
work within the same general vocational area might be
considered if the patient can accept the implied limitations.

Even within the old familiar environment, it may be necessary to restructure and simplify. For example, it would probably be best that a housewife returning home not be expected, at least initially, to handle the complexities of house management on her own.

MEMORY EFFECTS

One of the most common side effects of brain damage is some defect in memory. A fairly typical pattern, once the initial period of confusion lifts, is a complete blanking out of the time immediately surrounding the trauma. More serious and disturbing, however, is the continued inability of the patient to remember conversations, written material, telephone numbers, and sometimes faces, even for short periods of time. The loss of memory for the time of the illness and for new material may be so threatening that it may be psychologically necessary for the individual to develop defenses of denial and confabulation to protect himself. When a face, a time, an incident, is not remembered, the individual may "fake it." He may pretend to remember something and may even make up extensive and bizarre elaborations of the original memory to cover and establish his deception. He is not lying; he is desperately defending himself. We are all very dependent on our ability to retain information in order to function smoothly or at all in our complex society. Without this ability, an individual faces an almost completely novel challenge from one movement to the next without prior information and previous solutions. His life becomes like a series of disjointed movie still frames without the continuity that the memory factor provides. If, as is often the case, adaptive functioning is also adversely effected, the patient is in a fragile condition indeed.

Memory can be conveniently divided into three steps — intake, storage, and retrieval — and into two classes — language and spacial. If damage has occurred primarily to the left side of the brain, any memory loss may involve language, sequential reasoning, or numbers. For example, the individual may have trouble remembering telephone numbers even in the time between looking up the number and dialing. If the damage was primarily to the right side of the brain, visual/spacial memory aspects may predominate. Problems may be manifest in difficulties remembering directions, in recalling designs, or in reproducing two dimensional figures after a short delay. One of the more vivid examples of this kind of problem in the writer's experience involved a social worker. Immediately after her accident, she was unable to recall the faces of her clients although her memory for names, important aspects of the case, and relevant sequential planning had been relatively undiminished.

Available evidence suggests that the most typical deficit or difficulty following head injury occurs in the first step of the intake, storage, and retrieval sequence. Let us use a tape recorder analogy to illustrate what this means. The signal going into the machine may be weakened or distorted but once recorded, the *holding* and *replaying* aspects are relatively unaffected. Memory deficits may require special techniques to compensate for this intake problem. For example:

1. More repetitions of anything to be learned may be required.

2. Mechanical aides, i.e. lists, schedules, environmental structuring, concrete examples (such as simplifying and making as routine as possible the daily activities).

3. Use of memory extending techniques described in popular books and magazines such as *Psychology Today*, Sept., 1973.

4. Improvement of reading and study skills techniques to increase the availability and efficiency of the learning process.

For an individual in an intensive learning situation, such as a student going back into school, this process might involve several steps depending on the severity of the memory deficit. One program that has been useful for college students is as follows:

1. Auditing or taking at most one credit producing less for the first quarter of school. Simultaneous enrollment in any available reading and study skills improvement program.

2. Reduced load second quarter with a rigid schedule of study and work habit programming.

3. Third quarter load dependent on success in steps 1 and 2 and the degree of recovery.

TREATMENT AND RECOVERY

Medical

It is, of course, absolutely essential that the medical advice of your doctor be followed to the letter. Any damage to the brain can be a life-endangering condition and not one to be ignored or disregarded. Therapy and drug recommendations must be followed. Any radical change in the patient's thinking or emotional state should be reported since complications can reoccur. A sudden change may signal the onset of other problems.

Within the context of the medical treatment, however, natural recovery from most nonprogressive conditions often follows three definite steps following the trauma.

1. In the first six months, the acute phase of the illness passes and the most rapid recovery of all mental and physical functions occurs. This is undoubtedly the most important recovery period.

2. The second six months following the damage is still a period of recovery, but not as such a rapid rate.

3. The third and final six- to twelve-month period is one of slowed recovery and eventual stabilization. If proper treatment has been given throughout, residuals of physical, emotional, and cognitive limitations at the end of this time are unlikely to show great improvement.

Of all the stages discussed, the first is most important. Treatment delayed in initiation beyond this period will probably not be either as rapid nor as effective as immediate and intensive efforts. For example, many speech pathologists believe that the recovery rate of language function following any damage to the brain is twice as rapid in the first six months than in later periods. In consequence, if there are significant language problems, speak to your physician immediately as to his recommendations for speech therapy.

Other Treatment Possibilities

Speech: Speech therapists assist in the recovery of all language functioning, including not only articulation difficulties, but problems in the expression and understanding of speech, written and spoken. Their function and help is discussed at length in Chapter 4.

Occupational and physical therapy: Occupational and physical therapy on medical prescription can help the patient to recover his physical abilities and to prevent the deterioration of muscle tone and flexibility that can occur with the onset of stroke-induced paralysis. The treatments for the patient are exhausting, frustrating, and often painful; only the very motivated patient will wish to continue. The words, "He doesn't understand how hard it is," or "She's making me worse because I'm so tired," are so common in medical facilities as to be cliches. Sympathy and kindness seem to demand that we take the patient out of his program. But to be kind is not to be helpful, and sympathy is not always the same as love. To remove the patient prematurely and at his own wishes from the painful program may be to deprive him of more than optimal recovery of physical strength and range of motion; it may deprive him of something more critical, his self-respect.

Much of occupational therapy (O.T.) and physical therapy (P.T.) is oriented toward self-care skills and the Activities of Daily Living (A.D.L.). Simply stated, some measure of humanness that seems to be gone forever returns when one can relearn to shave or to button a shirt or to apply makeup, however badly. P.T. and O.T. are oriented toward the recovery of those mundane skills that mean so much when they are lost.

Emotional Support

Not all or even most of the effects of damage to the brain are dealt with by adjusting to the physical and mental limitations that may be there or even by relearning in an intensive rehabilitation unit. The initial reaction of the family of the stroke patient is shock and depression. Once the patient begins to recover, the family resources, personal and financial, are thrown into his support — to aid, to comfort, and to give what is necessary. But we are not talking about a period of hours, of days, or even weeks. Recovery is a matter of many months and may never be complete in the sense of return to full mental and physical strength. It becomes difficult to constantly adjust to the demands and needs of even someone deeply loved. Emotional controls may be lowered by the physical damage to the brain. The long period of time, the nagging fear of ultimate failure, and the sense of change within the patient begins to drain and erode even the closest family ties. The patient himself senses this, and coupled with his own anxieties and frustrations can become his own worst enemy, striking out verbally at those he loves most. No one likes complete dependence and no one enjoys the feeling of being a burden to his family. A descending spiral of distrust and anger can rip apart a marriage or a home that has endured many things before.

Before the psychological undercurrents become too strong, it would be better to anticipate the difficulties and to seek help from a pastor, a psychotherapist, or a social worker. Someone not directly involved but caring about what happens can often do a great deal to assist and to keep open rather than close the lines of communication.

Ultimately, if the family structure can no longer adjust and has been strained beyond the breaking point or if the patient's physical and mental state are beyond the capabilities of the home, the hard decision of nursing or convalescent home placement must be considered.

SOURCES OF HELP

The primary advisor for any major illness is the attending physician. He should be the first point of contact for any information you require. In addition the following agencies and professions may be invaluable to you.

Financial Aid

Serious illness is expensive, and if a vocation is interrupted, the financial pinch becomes even more acute. The following agencies may be of assistance:

1. Social welfare and social work services not only can be of direct assistance but are also experts in finding and utilizing other

community resources and services.

2. Vocational Rehabilitation can provide testing, therapy, and training if the case meets its criteria for eligibility and feasibility.

3. Easter Seal is another source of multidisciplinary services often at reduced or no cost.

4. Social Security has disability benefits but contact should be made early since there can be a considerable delay between application and assistance.

5. V.A. benefits may be available if the patient is a veteran, especially if extended care is needed.

Professional Services

Many of the following have been discussed in this chapter and can be found under their respective titles, under the general title "Rehabilitation" in the telephone book, in college or universities, or within most medical facilities:

1. Occupational therapy
2. Physical therapy
3. Psychologist
4. Speech pathologist
5. Neurologist
6. Veteran's assistance.

Chapter 2

STROKES

MOST people have known at one time or another someone who has suffered a stroke: a grandparent, an uncle, a father. The effects are usually profound and sudden and typically represent the most disturbing example of brain damage in the adult population.

DEFINITION

A stroke is basically a cutting off of the blood supply to the brain, usually on one side. The stopping of blood flow may be either caused by a blockage of a vessel or a rupture of that vessel. Since the brain more than any other organ must have oxygen to live, even a few moments of oxygen deprivation causes part of the brain to start to die. It is the death of the cells fed by the effected artery which causes the characteristic effects of stroke. Because the brain does not feel pain directly, the stroke may be painless and can even occur at night without waking the individual. The patient may awaken in the morning partially paralyzed, unable to speak, and totally confused.

The causes of stroke vary. A ruptured vessel can be caused by high blood pressure or some weakness of the wall of the vessel. A vessel may be blocked by deposits on the vessel wall (hardening of the arteries), a blood clot from another part of the body (heart or lungs), air, fat, or a clump of bacteria from a distant infection. Stroke is usually a disease of late middle age but can occur anytime if the patient has a congenital problem or if the individual uses drugs that can cause inflammation of the vessels. Usually the younger the individual the better his chances of recovery. The young often have vessels that can take over for the affected one.

In addition to the importance of age and general health in

recovery, the type and location of the stroke are critical. A hemorrhage is usually more dangerous than a blockage (emboli, thrombosis) because the escaping blood can cause its own damage by taking up space in the skulls and by directly destroying brain cells. Location of the damage is important because the artery system that supplies the brain looks like a tree with a thick trunk and gradually smaller and smaller limbs and branches. Damage to a vessel effects all the smaller vessels that come from it. The higher in the arterial tree, the smaller the vessels and the less extensive the brain area effected by the damage to the system.

The brain is divided into left and right sides. Each side controls the opposite side of the body and involves different thinking processes. Since usually only one side of the brain (hemisphere) is effected by a stroke, what happens to the patient depends on which side is damaged. Which hemisphere is damaged is usually easily seen by the characteristic paralysis on one side of the body. If the left hemisphere is damaged, some part of the right side of the body is effected. If the right hemisphere is effected, the left side of the body is influenced. The sudden inability of the patient to control or even feel an arm and a leg, the characteristic droop of the facial muscles, and the slurred or absent speech can both disturb and repel.

Because of the extent and the often sharply defined area of damage to the brain, much of what could be said about strokes is discussed in Chapter 1. When an individual has a stroke to the left hemisphere, he will often have most of the possible symptoms put down under the "Left Hemisphere," "Memory," and "Adaptive" sections of Chapter 1. Right hemisphere stroke includes much of "Right Hemisphere," "Memory," and "Adaptive" sections of Chapter 1. To review, however, the next few paragraphs will outline stroke effects.

The effects of stroke to each side could be outlined as follows:
I. Left Hemisphere Stroke (see "Left Hemisphere" section of Chapter 1)
    A. Right side weakness or paralysis
    B. Right side insensitivity to touch or even pain
    C. Disruption of language (see "Aphasia" chapter)
    D. Memory disturbances (see Ch. 1 on "Memory Effects,"

especially language memory)
E. Adaptive functioning damaged (see Ch. 1)
F. Inability to see in the right visual field of each eye may occur

II. Right Hemisphere Stroke (see "Right Hemisphere" section of Chapter 1)
A. Left side weakness or paralysis
B. Right side insensitivity to touch
C. Disruption of spatial abilities (see Ch. 1)
D. Memory disturbances (see spatial memory in Ch. 1)
E. Adaptive functioning often sharply curtailed but sometimes masked by intact language in a structural setting
F. Inability to see in the left visual field of both eyes can happen

Because a stroke usually does considerable damage to one hemisphere or the other, most of the characteristics outlined above under the appropriate side can be present at least early in the recovery picture (see Ch. 1).

To illustrate more fully the effects, personal and psychological, of a stroke, the following case write-up may be helpful. If the technical language becomes confusing, read only the recommendations section. Unlike most stroke patients, this individual is a young housewife. Her stroke is to the left and fairly small in area. She is presently employed following treatment. The complete technical report is in the appendix.

Age: 32   Agency: Residential Program

REFERRAL INFORMATION: Mrs. A suffered a stroke two years ago and has since entered the Residential Program. The neuropsychological examination was requested to assess her recovery to this point, her present level of functioning, and potential for further recovery. A previous administration of the Reitan Neuropsychological Battery was conducted six-and-a-half months ago, permitting a close comparison of test findings to assess recovery.

TESTS ADMINISTERED:
Reitan Neuropsychological Battery

Wechsler Adult Intelligence Scale — WAIS
Aphasia Screening Test
Category Test
Word Finding Test
Trail Marking Test — Parts A & B
Tactual Performance Test — TPT
Seashore Rhythm Test
Speech Sounds Perception Test
Hand Dynamometer
Finger Oscillation Test

GENERAL OBSERVATIONS: Testing was conducted over a two-day period and proceeded with no major difficulties. Mrs. A was quite anxious at the beginning of the first session, but soon became relaxed and talked more freely with this examiner. She recalled the session with a psychologist at another clinic which the examiner had attended over six months ago. The previous contact with this examiner seemed to help her relax in the present situation.

Although apparently comfortable and relaxed throughout both sessions, she frequently showed signs of an expressive dysphasia through marked hesitancy in speaking and occasional forgetting of names, places, and events from her past. This feature of her interaction with the examiner was a source of embarrassment for Mrs. A, but one which she handled well overall. Throughout both sessions she seemed to put forth her best effort to perform on the tests and did not seem threatened by the possibility of failure. This may in part reflect her previous exposure to the Battery.

TESTS RESULTS AND INTERPRETATIONS: Tests of biological intelligence yielded an Impairment Index of .57, indicating a mild impairment of adaptive abilities dependent on organic brain functioning. Performance on the Seashore Rhythm Test and the Speech Sounds Perception Test was in the brain damaged range for both. This would suggest difficulty in correctly perceiving and integrating auditory stimuli in situations which involve fine discriminations. The location score of the TPT fell into the brain damaged range. The Finger Oscillation Test showed slightly impaired performance with the preferred hand, but not enough to constitute a burden in day-to-day living.

Tests of psychometric intelligence revealed the following. On the Wechsler Adult Intelligence test, she scored in the Normal Range overall, but Verbal IQ fell into the Borderline Range, twenty-eight points lower than her Normal Performance IQ. Such a wide range of performance on the WAIS is uncommon for normal individuals and is likely a result of the brain damage. Her score on the Word Finding Test also was less than average. This would tend to indicate some impairment of reasoning and verbal problem-solving ability.

On the Aphasia Screening Test, there was consistent evidence of dysnomia, dyslexia, central dysarthria, and mild dyscalculia. There was also evidence of right-left confusion. On the Sensory-Perceptual portion of the test, Tactile and Visual perception were normal, but three errors in Auditory perception occurred with the left ear on double simultaneous stimulation. Dystereognosis was observed from her misperceiving a coin placed in the right hand five out of six trials and two out of six trials with the left hand.

In summary, the pattern of test scores constitutes mild impairment of biological and psychometric intelligence. The brain damage seems to be mainly localized to the left hemisphere and appears to be highly focal in nature, including the anterior temporal area, extending anteriorly into the parietal area. It is difficult to rule out any right hemisphere involvement on the basis of the tests administered, but the comparison of hemispheres seems to point out maximal involvement of the left hemisphere.

Before discussing recovery and the potential for improvement, it is worthwhile to look at previous performance. Starting with biological intelligence, there is improvement in several areas. Finger oscillation went from 20 with the preferred hand to 49, and from 30 to 39 with the nonpreferred hand. On the TPT, the times overall are relatively unchanged; however, her relative performance with both hands has improved relative to use of each hand alone. Her Memory score went from 7 to 9, both in the normal range, but the location score went from a normal 5 to an impaired 3 on the second administration. Random fluctuation and/or temporary confusion and anxiety may account for the latter result. The error score on the Category Test went from 95 to 28, but this test can be sensitive to bias when administered twice to the same person, especially someone with a relatively intact long-term memory. It is difficult to say just how much of the difference is due to recovery and how much is due to bias. The overall Impairment Index was unchanged from the first to the second administration with the improvement on Category Test being cancelled out by the poorer Location score for the TPT. Therefore, adaptive abilities based on organic brain functioning have remained at a level of mild impairment.

On the WAIS, the overall scores were relatively unchanged. Verbal IQ score went from 84 to 78, Performance IQ score increased from 99 to 106, and the Full Scale IQ score increased from 99 to 106, and the Full Scale IQ of 90 was unchanged. Since the WAIS was administered at the beginning of the first session by this examiner, temporary uneasiness may have contributed to the lower Verbal IQ score, but not enough to alter greatly the test results. On the inspection of individual subtests, the most noticeable difference was on Digit Span, improving from a scaled score of 1 to a score of 6, indicating some improvement in the area of short-term memory. Otherwise, in psychometric intelligence there was no significant change from the previous level.

Qualitatively, the Aphasia Screening Test showed an amelioration of the dysphasic symptoms from the prior examination until this examination. The same pattern of deficits, however, appears on both examinations. The Sensory-Perceptual portion of this test also revealed the presence of dystereognosis on both occasions with no apparent change. There was no indication of auditory suppression on earlier examination.

Mrs. A has suffered some loss of abilities because of the stroke but has recovered to a large extent. The damage to the brain was on the left side in the language centers, and the problems which remain are primarily in language processing verbal intelligence has been lowered, adaptive reasoning has been decreased, and reading and writing skills have been influenced. In ordinary conversation, Mrs. A would have little difficulty, but if she is tired, is bombarded on all sides by sounds, or must follow a long, complicated set of directions, she is impaired.

In the time since her last testing Mrs. A has shown good improvement, especially in the ability to "think on her feet." Her memory for spatial and language is almost at a normal level, and she shows fine recovery of language/communication abilities. Coordination, strength, and speed are all up, but not to completely unimpaired levels.

Recovery, judging from past testing, seems to be stable. Significant improvement in important abilities has occurred. Since Mrs. A has received little therapy for her speech and reading problem, further improvement in these important areas is possible.

RECOMMENDATIONS

Returning now to the question of recovery and further potential for improvement, the following conclusions seem reasonable. The patient's condition has been relatively stable over the past six months in regard to overall levels of psychometric and biological intelligence. There has been an observable reduction in dysphasic symptoms, a slight improvement on tasks requiring simple and complex motor movements. Performance in that latter area, however, still remains in the impaired range of functioning. Although one cannot rule out completely the possibility of some additional recovery of function to premorbid levels, based on her age and number of months posttrauma, such improvement would likely be less rapid. Based on the relative lack of intensive therapy prior to entry into the Program, one could expect additional improvement in the area of language skills, i.e. reading and speaking.

As for self-help skills and resumption of everyday activities after completion of the Program, the overall pattern of test results indicates near normal to normal levels of ability in most areas relevant to adaptive functioning. Although one might expect some slowness in complex motor tasks and slight difficulties with reacting to novel situations which require quick, integrative problem solving, these do not seem like great enough obstacles to interfere with carrying out of household duties and/or the successful performance in a job situation. Looking more closely, she is capable of holding a job which does not emphasize contact with people (such as a sales clerk) or demand integrative thinking, abstraction, or problem solving as the emphasis of the job. Judging from her motivation to perform on the tests and her overall interest in her own rehabilitation, it seems that she would be well motivated to perform in further rehabilitative efforts or a job setting. As for her emotional needs, this examiner feels that being able to be with her family again and finding a job which affords some contact with people along with a supportive employer are important factors to consider in helping her readjust to everyday life.

Chapter 3

HEAD INJURIES

SERIOUS blows to the head can occur at any age. Although many serious neurological conditions (tumors, strokes, hardening of the arteries, etc.) are more likely to occur above the age of forty, car crashes, bike accidents, and sport accidents can abruptly change the life of the healthiest, most active child or young adult.

Definition

A serious blow to the head may or may not involve actual physical penetration of the skull. Cracking of the protective bone at the site of the injury and bruising of underlying tissue may occur. Unconsciousness, sometimes for extended periods of time; varying periods of confusion; memory loss; and headaches are common side effects of the injury. Personality changes can occur if the blow is a serious one.

BEHAVIORAL EFFECTS

The effects of a severe head injury are complex. The damage and effects are not necessarily confined to the site of the blow. The brain of man, although delicate and complex, fortunately is well packaged against injury. It is protected not only by the tough bone of the skull, but is is also covered by layers of tough membrane and is suspended in fluid. Liquid within and around the brain can spread out and dampen the effects of a blow. We can all remember being accidently hit on the head as children, usually with no more effect than a headache or a superficial scar or two. Considering the delicacy of brain tissue, the inability of brain tissue to regenerate, and the number of accidents sustained, the usual minimal effects of head injuries are remarkable indeed.

21

When significant trauma damage to the brain does occur, the behavioral effects are complex. It cannot be assumed, for example, that damage to the right of the head influences only the right side of the brain and its functions. At the site of the blow, damage to underlying vessels may produce hemorrhage and blood clots. Brain swelling (edema) may occur and produce its own effects through pressure.

Some of the force of the original blow can be transmitted through the brain and produce secondary damage to the other side. If bone, dirt, or foreign body particles penetrate the skull cavity, the possibility of a generalized or local infection of the brain can also occur. Surgery with its own characteristic side effects may be necessary to save the life of the individual. Usually the whole brain is effected, one side more than the other. When actual penetration of the skull occurs, it is far more likely that damage will be mostly in one hemisphere. The reader may find rereading those parts of Chapter 1 which deal with the site of the injury (right or left) helpful. Remember, however, that usually head trauma involves damage to both sides of the brain, one side more than the other. Because of this effect, some lesser effects from damage to the opposite side of the brain may influence and complicate the picture.

RECOVERY

Typically the period of unconsciousness that may follow an accident is one index of severity. A blow occurs at a given moment and then stops. The injury that happens then begins to show improvement (medical and psychological) over time. The more recent the accident, the worse the patient looks. The patient begins getting better rather than worse as in some progressive neurological conditions, i.e. tumors or multiple sclerosis.

Although recovery potential is actually an extremely positive aspect of head injuries, the family may not realize the patient will improve. Head injuries typically have an acute phase in which the patient is most obviously medically effected. There may be a period of unconsciousness, sometimes of substantial duration (days or weeks); confusion alternating with lucid moments, memory gaps, partial paralysis, and obvious cognitive effects in language, reasoning, and ability. When the patient is no longer so obviously in danger and no longer relatively unaware of his limitations, a period of depression and outright fear can occur, especially if some physical residuals or seizures remain after the accident. For example, the voluntary control of muscles is second nature to us. Striking a match, opening a door, maintaining an erect posture are acts we don't think or worry about until we can no longer perform them smoothly or at will (see Ch. 6). Even more traumatic is the presence of seizures as a result of the accident. Seizures frighten: the loss of consciousness, the jerking spasms, the abrupt loss of bowel and bladder control that may go along with a seizure are strange and repelling. Seizures can occur on a limited or on a permanent basis up to one year after a severe blow to the head. They can usually be medically controlled with proper treatment. Since seizures may occur in many neurological conditions, a separate chapter is devoted to them (see Ch. 5).

At that moment of realization of loss — days, weeks, or even months after the accident — the patient is at his worst medically and psychologically. Without knowledge of the recovery potential he may feel that he is always going to be as "bad" as he is now. The recently injured college student unable to understand or remember the meaning of a single line from a textbook who believes that he will always have such a deficit has reason, indeed, to be anxious, upset, and hostile.

No one can predict the exact rate or ultimate extent of recovery from a head injury. Broad generalizations can be made but they may not hold in the individual case.

1. Usually the young individual recovers most rapidly and completely. This is fortunate since the young have a gift for getting themselves into physically damaging accidents in the first place.

2. The seriousness and extent of the original damage is also an obvious variable. Your doctor is the proper source of information in this area.

3. Other factors that can be mentioned but probably are of limited practical assistance to the family are the general health of the patient, his abilities before the accident, side effects associated

with the injury (i.e. infection, necessary surgical intervention).

4. The seriousness of any deficit, mental or physical, depends on what the individual is asked to do in the outside world. The "fit" of the damage that remains and the job or school of the patient are critical in determining the seriousness of the loss and to some extent the probable emotional response to the loss.

It is, of course, absolutely essential that the medical advice of your doctor be followed to the letter. The mechanism of severe closed head injury can be a life-endangering condition and not one to be ignored or disregarded. Therapy and drug recommendations must be followed. Any radical change in the patient's thinking or emotional state should be reported since complications can occur and be signaled by a sudden shift in behavior.

Within the context of the medical treatment, however, natural recovery seems to follow three definite steps following the trauma.

1. The first six months in which the acute phase of the illness passes and the most rapid recovery of all mental and physical functions occurs. This is undoubtedly the most important recovery period.

2. The second six months following the trauma is still a period of recovery, but not at such a rapid rate.

3. The third and final twelve- to eighteen-month period is one of slowed recovery and eventual stabilization. If proper treatment has been given throughout, residuals of physical, emotional, and cognitive limitations at the end of this time are unlikely to show further improvement.

Of all stages discussed, the first is most important from a recovery standpoint. Treatment delayed in initiation beyond this period will probably not be either as rapid or as effective as immediate and intensive efforts. For example, many speech pathologists believe that the recovery rate of language function following any damage to the brain is twice as effective in the first six months as in later periods. In consequence, if there are significant language problems, speak to your physician immediately as to his recommendations for speech therapy (see chapter on aphasia).

EMOTIONAL EFFECTS

The emotional consequences of a severe blow to the head often go beyond the natural depression and sense of loss to be expected when any serious illness occurs. Sometimes as a direct medical consequence of the damage to the brain, the patient may experience severe shifts in his normal emotional makeup. These shifts might be described as a lowering of the emotional control factor and a decrease, sometimes substantial, in emotional stability of the patient. The individual may change from a calm, placid person to one alternating unexpectedly between bleak depression and flaring anger. The patient can shift widely and abruptly without warning. Two case studies may illustrate the problem.

John Smith, a high school junior and star athlete, was injured following a severe blow to the head in a game. To prevent further injury and to insure his safety, he sat on the bench for the rest of the season. Although without a record before the accident, he began to create a long list of difficulties with the police including reckless driving, driving while intoxicated, simple assault, and petty theft, all impulsive, poorly considered acts. He finally dropped out of school before graduating.

Rex Brown, a college junior, was in a car accident that almost took his life. Upon returning to school after recovering, he noticed several disturbing changes, including impulsive anger. Although a mild and gentle individual, he found that he had increasing trouble controlling his temper. Following a class in which one of his classmates repeatedly ridiculed the instructor, Rex walked up to the classmate and knocked him over several seats. Because of Rex's good record, his punishment was minimal and he continued in school.

Often, medical assistance, medication, careful programming, and the natural recovery function are sufficient to bring about a suitable return to normal control. However, psychiatric or psychological assistance for both the patient and his family may be necessary to help them to adjust and to understand why the patient sometimes acts in an irrational or irresponsible way. To illustrate the usual effects of a closed head injury, the following formal case may be helpful. If the technical language of the report interferes with understanding, refer to the Summary section.

Chronological Age: 20-11   Grade in School: Junior in college

TESTS ADMINISTERED:
Complete Neuropsychological Battery (Reitan)
    Trails A & B — Halstead Category Test
    Strength of Grip (Dynamometer)
    Minnesota Multiphasic Personality Inventory
    Wechsler Adult Intelligence Scale
    Seashore Rhythm Test
    Speech Perception Test
    Wepman-Halstead Aphasia Screening Test
    Complete Audiological Evaluation

PRESENTING PROBLEM: This young college student was in a severe motorcycle accident last summer, followed by a two-week period of unconsciousness. He is concerned about his recovery progress and when he will be able to return to school, as well as when it will be possible for him to drive.

PREVIOUS TESTING PERFORMED: Patient indicated that several neurological examinations had been completed.

OBSERVATIONS OF BEHAVIOR: The patient was neat and well-dressed for both examination periods. He had indicated his willingness to undergo the extensive eight-hour testing period and maintained good rapport with the examiner. He was very concerned about several of the tests, and questions such as "What is this supposed to prove?", "What do you find out from this?", were very frequent. The examiner attributed this to his anxiety about the outcome of the test results, and whenever possible, was answered very directly and honestly. This appears to be appreciated by the patient, and the questioning subsided during the last part of the testing.

INTERPRETATION: In terms of intellectual functioning, there is probably a depression on the Verbal IQ score, primarily because of a very low-digit span subtest. The motoric problems become obvious on the performance items of the WAIS. Lower scores on these test items (involving sequencing) depress the Performance IQ. The client was very pleased that he was able to do well on the

Block Design section. He remembered doing these right after the accident, with very poor results. There is a remarkable sparing of higher level adaptive functioning and indications of excellent recovery potential. WAIS answers were good, but quality of answers may still be slightly depressed.

The good levels of adaptation and abstraction for learning were supported by the strong showing on the Halstead Category Test. The machine was malfunctioning on that day, and the examiner often had to resort to verbal reinforcement which could be very confusing under the best of conditions. This was handled well by him, and his scores improved on each subtest in spite of the confusion produced by testing procedures.

However, where problem solving also involved sequencing, as on the Trails Test A and B, he had more difficulty. Even though there were three trials prior to Test B, he had obvious difficulty in going from letters to numbers and in extending his anticipatory set.

Motoric problems showed up on the writing items of the Wepman (associated in part, probably, with reported visual field problems), the slow performance on the Tactual Performance Test with the right hand, and the obvious slowdown in Strength of Grip and Finger Tapping scores for the right hand.

The large number of errors on the Speech Perception Test (SPT) prompted the examiner to request the Audiological Examination. Most errors on the SPT were on higher frequency sounds, such as th and f. As indicated from the Hearing Test results, his hearing is well within normal limits.

Although the client had no difficulty with the Visual Section of the Wepman Screening, he indicated that his field is narrowed for finer movements in both eyes, suggestive of a right hemianopsia. Astereognosis was indicated for the right hand, with some limited responses as well as on the Fingertip Number Writing Perception; again with the right hand.

SUMMARY COMMENTS: Higher level functioning is maintained well, with minimal sensory damage and some speech perception problems in evidence. Recovery has been remarkable, especially in view of the fact that it has not yet been six months since the accident. Good recovery potential is indicated.

The sequencing, motor control, and vision problems present

difficulties, and driving would not be recommended at this time.

Test results indicate primarily left hemisphere dysfunction with some motoric problems. Overall Impairment Index score for the complete battery would be .6 (on a 1.0 scale) suggesting "mild brain damage" category.

P.T. and O.T. may be helpful with finer hand movements and training in working with both hands. The minimal dysarthric qualities in his speech he feels do not need attention. He stressed the fact that he spoke slowly before the accident and that his stress and intonation patterns were also much the same as now. He also mentioned that his speech has improved significantly since the accident.

Retesting in four to six months may indicate the continuing improvement in overall scores.

SUMMARY AND RECOMMENDATIONS

Injuries from blows to the head are common, especially in the young. The pattern of difficulties, physical and reasoning, that occurs vary, but may include
1. memory problems
2. emotional volitility
3. speech and language problems
4. seizures

The recovery of the individual from his injury can take as long as three years and can be assisted by proper treatment including (as needed)
1. speech therapy
2. occupational and physical therapy
3. psychology or psychiatry
4. neurology

Chapter 4

APHASIA

GENERAL DEFINITION

THE ability to express and receive written and spoken language represents one of man's most fundamental and important achievements. Language is the basis for communication with others, the shorthand of the thinking processes, and the mirror of intelligence and personality. The failure of language to develop because of brain damage or the disruption of established language abilities because of damage to the brain is *aphasia*.

For most of mankind, the left side of the brain (hemisphere) is the center of language. Some cases have been reported of limited language ability in adults after complete removal of the left hemisphere, but they are rare. For very young children and for left-handed adults, the picture is less clear, but generally speaking, significant damage to the left side of the brain from accident, disease, or both can often lead to aphasia.

Severity

There are many useful ways of describing and categorizing aphasia. Among the simpler dimensions are severity and type. Severity can range broadly. Global aphasia, for example, is the most complete. Global aphasia means that most major language abilities are severely impaired. The individual cannot speak or even understand simple directions. Such an individual would be unable to communicate his simplest ideas or to understand directions even at the level of "close the door" or "point to the chair." At the other end of the severity continuum, language disruption could be limited to a momentary inability to find precisely the right word without a delay. For example, "That's a . . . . chair." It might be noted that everyone can display such mild difficulties when fatigued or intoxicated.

Type

A useful way of understanding aphasia is to use the two categories of *receptive* (sensory) and *expressive* (motor). Although the two categories overlap and rarely occur in isolation, it is obvious that in using language, we are either sending out something (expressive) or receiving something (receptive). We are either using our own words (expressive) or understanding someone else's words or symbols (receptive).

Receptive Aphasia

Receptive aphasia involves an inability to translate or understand language or other symbols (since numbers must be translated too) written or spoken to us. Receptive language abilities are probably more fundamental and necessary to the individual and will be discussed first.

It has been found that the expressive abilities can vary greatly in development, depending on culture and environment. Receptive abilities however, at least in the earliest years, seem to follow the same pattern and rate despite differences in country of origin and home environment. This patterning assumes, however, relatively normal (within broad limits) nutrition, health, and educational stimulation.

The names associated with the various kinds of receptive/ expressive aphasias are impressive, but most are fairly easy to understand once described and illustrated. Accordingly, major kinds of aphasias will be described and examples of each will be given to clarify the description. The descriptions and examples are given to clarify and translate the bewildering professional jargon into something approximating the English language.

Visual Form Agnosia: Nothing is implied in this aphasia about the ability of the eyes to see. Vision itself is not affected. The individual is simply unable to attach the correct verbal label to some simple abstract form that he sees. For example, when shown a triangle he may hesitate, be unable to reply, or may call it something else, i.e. a box. He still sees the form, can still trace or draw its shape, but cannot come up with the right word for it.

Visual Letter Agnosia: This condition is similar to visual form agnosia but is more specific in its effects. The individual cannot correctly or reliably label all the letters of the alphabet. He may completely fail to read the letter, may substitute another letter for it, or may just delay a long time before giving the correct response.

Alexia or Dyslexia: In this condition the individual's ability to read is diminished or even completely taken away. For example, a person who completed high school may find himself unable to read a newspaper following a stroke, even though the newspaper is written at a comparatively simple word level. Dyslexia in children is covered in Chapter 7 as *Minimal Brain Damage.*

Auditory Verbal Agnosia: In this condition, the individual is exposed to some spoken langauge; he hears the sounds but is unable to comprehend the meaning of the word, i.e. when given the command, "close the door," the individual may look frustrated, signal his attention nonverbally, but be unable to comply completely with one request. He hears, but he does not understand.

Auditory Number Agnosia: In this highly selective condition, the individual hears numbers spoken or read to him but is unable to understand their meaning, magnitude, or relationship to each other. If the individual has often worked with numbers, i.e. an accountant, salesperson, or waitress, such a failure is very threatening.

Expressive Aphasias

Expressive abilities involve those skills utilized when the individual produces or expresses some written or oral communication. These are the skills evident when we write, spell, or name things. Such abilities are probably more dependent on educational and environmental factors than are receptive abilities.

Anomia or Disnomia: This kind of aphasia is evident when the individual has difficulty in attaching labels to common objects.

For example, when shown a picture of a clock, he may be unable to name the object, may substitute another word or group of words for the precise name, or may hesitate for a long time before answering. With individuals who normally have a good vocabulary or verbal facility, another defense or reaction to the anomia may appear, circumlocution. Circumlocution is the psychological way of coping involved when an individual discovers his difficulty in finding the single word or phrase that the situation requires. If the single word is not available to him, he talks around the word and describes it. For example, when shown the picture of a clock, he may say, "Uh, that is the round thing that goes around and tells time and has two hands." The example is an extreme case but does illustrate the behavior.

Spelling Apraxia: Disruption of the individual's normal ability to spell is spelling apraxia. Since spelling skills vary tremendously depending on educational and individual factors, the presence or absence of this condition is sometimes a matter of judgment. However, the person who has had twelve years of education who is unable to spell "square" has probably lost some skills in this area.

Agraphia: The ability to write in at least a minimally legible fashion is necessary for written communication. When an individual shows a sharp decrement in his ability to write because of damage to the brain, the condition is called *agraphia*. Often, the writing produced is characterized by not only irregular and angular strokes but also may show a characteristic called *perseveration*. In this context, perseveration may be considered present if the individual continues a movement when it should stop. For example, "n's" and "m's" may be written with too many humps, and individual letters may be repeated several times in the middle of words.

Childhood Aphasia

Learning to speak and to understand speech is one of the great accomplishments of anyone's life. Because the process is usually so smooth and expected, this great feat of learning is ignored and taken for granted after the milestone of the first word. But the coding, abstracting, perceiving process that we call language is complicated and can be slowed, interrupted, and stopped by a variety of conditions including brain damage, mental retardation, deafness, emotional disturbance, and environmental factors. When language, receptive or expressive, is delayed or stopped in development because of damage or congenital factors of the brain, the condition is called *childhood aphasia*. Before the diagnosis of childhood aphasia can be made however, the following possible causes of arrested speech and language must be ruled out.

1. *Mental Retardation*: A child's absent or limited speech may be more in accord with his mental abilities than his chronological age.

2. *Mental Disturbance*: A psychotic child can show extremes of language impairment. He may be totally mute. He may show bewildering variability (a child may vary in language usage from infant level to well above chronological age). There may be echolalia when the child does not initiate or use spontaneous appropriate speech but rather parrots the words he hears around him. Such a child when asked, "What is your name?" might reply, "What is your name?"

3. *Sensory Loss:* The child with a hearing loss, complete or partial, may show speech delay. The child may respond to noise but can not discriminate the critical elements of speech. His condition may be masked by such selective hearing loss.

4. *Environmental Deprivation*: At least some minimal exposure at home to common objects and speech is necessary for the usual development of speech whether dialect or standard.

Although children may speak their first word at nine or ten months and generally can follow very simple commands by one year, there is considerable variability in normal children in the development and acquisition of speech. In addition, many factors operating by themselves or in combination can delay or stop language. Not all delayed speech is aphasia. Typically, finding out the cause of delayed speech is a complicated process, sometimes requiring the efforts of many disciplines like physicians, audiologists, speech pathologists, and psychologists. But without knowledge of the underlying cause, proper treatment is impossible. The physician in charge of a case represents the coordinating and referring person at the center of the complex diagnostic process.

Unintelligible Speech

In addition to the expressive and receptive difficulties described above, speech may not be intelligible. Three major conditions are described:

1. Childhood articulation difficulties may involve delayed development (when the youngster's speech resemble that of a younger child), substitutions of sounds, and other problems.

2. Dysarthria involves difficulty in the rapid movement of the muscles of speech sometimes including paralysis of those muscles. Speech is slurred.

3. Dyspraxia of speech is an inability to coordinate smoothly the individual movements of speech. Single muscle movements may be unaffected but sequencing of the movements breaks down. For example the individual may be unable to start a word, but can complete the sequence if prompted with the first sound.

SPEECH PATHOLOGY

Speech pathologists and speech therapists are trained to work with children and adults who have communication disorders. The range of ages and presenting problems in their caseload is wide. They may work with any problem from mild articulation problems in young children to profound aphasia in the aged. Speech pathologists often work closely with physicians, audiologists, and psychologists since medical, hearing, and psychological factors can be of great importance in any diagnostic or therapeutic workup.

Generally speaking, before speech therapy begins, the speech pathologist will test and interview to determine the nature and extent of the problem. This diagnostic part of therapy will vary in time from a few minutes to several hours, depending on the complexity of the communication problem. The diagnostic process is often complicated, and it may be necessary to bring in other disciplines to assist. However, without some idea of the causes and extent of the problem, it is difficult to set up an effective and precise treatment plan. Usually, once the diagnosis has been completed, the results are communicated to the family or to the referring physician. Treatment, if needed, can then begin.

Treatment is usually at least weekly, although this can vary from less than once a week to several times a week depending on the patient's needs and availability of therapists. The exact nature of treatment for any given individual will also vary depending on his needs and age.

As with many rehabilitation treatments, the patient's motivation to continue is necessary, but often difficult to maintain. Programs may seem tedious and childish, especially if the treatment involves a great deal of drill. Sometimes adults become incensed because their program must begin at the present communication level rather than their previously highest skill. For example, after a stroke it is possible that even the most highly educated individual may show signs of dysnomia (difficulty in naming objects on demand). One task that might begin treatment would be to show pictures of common objects (i.e. toothbrush) and ask the person to name it. Typically, the speech pathologist will begin with the strongest language areas retained and work to the weaker. Even so, a former engineer asked to name a toothbrush and unable to do so will feel angry and frustrated. The patient may feel that the therapist is treating him like a child and playing silly games. Coupled with the natural frustration of adjusting to his new and disturbing limitations, the negative feelings of the patient toward therapy may cause him to wish to withdraw impulsively from treatment. Before the patient's feelings get to this point, the patient and his family should talk frankly and honestly with the therapist. A speech therapist has worked with many difficult problems and can be of great assistance in the adjustment to the tedium of therapy. But the therapist can only help if he knows what is going on. As much as he would like to, the therapist cannot read minds and can only respond to what he sees and hears. Again, before any radical decisions are made to discontinue treatment, the patient and family should at least talk about their feelings. Speech threapy can help, often in very difficult cases, but only if the patient stays in treatment as recommended. This is especially true in cases of aphasia since not only the nature and extent of therapy are important but also its timing. Recovery is often dependent on intensive work at the right time.

However, even with the highest motivation, a good treatment program, and good rapport between patient and therapist, great variability of performance will occur. The patient may, on a given day, be unable to do or say something he could do easily the day before. Such variability is expected by the therapist, but even for her the sudden (and temporary) decrease in performance is frustrating. For the patient and his family, an abrupt difficulty can be frightening.

Some of this variability in therapy cannot be accounted for. The abrupt increases and decreases in performance are like the good and bad days that every one has but are more extreme. Since they cannot be predicted or controlled, there is little need to be concerned about these day-to-day variations. They will occur and typically will not disrupt the process of therapy.

Some variability effects can be noted and controlled. When fatigue, alcohol, or emotional disturbances reach a certain point in all of us, our thinking processes and to some extent, our speech, are effected. We stutter, search for words, slur our speech, and in general display many of the behavioral characteristics of asphasics. True aphasics are closer to this disruptive edge than other people. For example, even fairly mild drinking can cause an aphasic patient for a short time to display many of the symptoms that had disappeared with time and treatment. Even a patient with good recovery and no noticeable speech residuals can have a little trouble with language at the end of a fatiguing day.

One short precautionary note. When a patient displays very abrupt changes in language, thinking, or emotional responses, they must be communicated to the therapist or the physician, since the change may signal a shift in the medical picture. Day-to-day variation is expected, but extreme breaks in the normal pattern of behavior may indicate trouble that must be dealt with medically.

Two cases are presented here to illustrate this confusing

condition of aphasia. Case #1 shows a typical pattern of language difficulties following a severe head injury and illustrates the problems of readjustment to school.

TESTS ADMINISTERED: Full Reitan Battery, including the WAIS and MMPI; Suicide Potential Scale; Wide Range Achievement Test.

PRESENTING PROBLEM: This twenty-one-year-old Caucasion male was referred to the clinic for a complete intellectual, psychological, and organic evaluation of his current level of functioning.

While driving last spring, he was involved in a serious two-car accident. He was admitted to the hospital with facial lacerations and "left temporal lobe contusion." The admitting doctor noticed less movement in the right extremities and a right facial lag; subsequently, he was transferred to another hospital for a complete neurological workup. Tracheotomy, arteriogram, lumbar punctures, and a left temporal decompression were performed, and he was discharged in May, with a prognosis of "fair." There is a residual right paresis (hemi), mild spastic dysarthria, and the patient is wearing a partial brace on the right leg which goes up to the knee.

PREVIOUS TESTING PERFORMED: At the time of initial testing, the patient was enrolled for therapy and was being seen for physical therapy, occupational therapy, and speech therapy. The Porch Index for Communicative Abilities (a test for aphasia) had been administered, with findings of mild spastic dysarthria and mild anomia.

OBSERVATION OF BEHAVIOR: The patient was always most cooperative during the extensive testing over the two days, but appeared extremely anxious about his condition. Statements such as "The doctor said I'd get better, but I'm not" were typical. He was very concerned about whether his answers were correct, or whether his performance time was good. On tests that involved his affected arm, he was particularly anxious. During the Tactual Performance Test (the patient was blindfolded throughout), he refused more than one rest period when using his right hand. Since this test took almost twice as long as normal, the muscle tension became evident by the appearance of a slight tremor of the head and left hand. He became dizzy after the completion of this test and rested for about fifteen minutes, complaining of vision problems.

Several times during both periods of testing, he mentioned his feelings of depression and his thoughts of suicide. "I know I'll never do it, but I think about it a lot," was a typical statement.

His speech causes him anxiety, although articulation is good. He feels "like a lot of saliva is in my mouth — it's like mush," and expressed his resentment that he could not talk fast "like I used to" without slurring words. Although in speech therapy, the therapist reports he has only appeared one time out of the three scheduled to this date. He appeared obviously impatient with his speech "It's not improving."

The depressed state of the client during the second testing period and his reference several times to suicide prompted the examiner to have a neuropsychologist see the patient at that time. The doctor spoke with the patient for a short while, explaining that opportunities would be available for him to see someone to talk to about his immediate concerns about his depression. At this time, he indicated that he was becoming very interested in astrology and felt that the state of the world was due to the fact that society had ignored the study of the stars and astrological signs.

The WAIS performance agitated the patient, apparently because he needed constant reassurance as to whether he had given the right answer. Encouragement during the latter part of the test when he performed well brought forth comments from the client such as "big deal!" Self-deprecation, while only occasionally mentioned by the client during testing, was much more evident during this test.

INTERPRETATION: *Intellectual functioning* — On the basis of the WAIS findings, he would have a difficult time performing at a college level. The difficulties with anomia (word-finding) and language may possibly not improve due to the time that has elapsed since the accident without therapy. The Category test and Tactual Performance test indicate a lack of spatial orientation and judgment, plus inability for short-term recall of learning. The definite paresis is a factor in motoric performance for the right hand, which was his dominant hand prior to the accident.

Emotional functioning — Prior to the accident, he was

reported to be losing weight, eating improperly, and not sleeping well. This information was noted in the medical records upon admittance to the hospital immediately after the accident.

Between test periods, the patient related to the examiner that prior to his accident he had been taking mescaline, LSD, marihuana, speed, and other hallucogenics. His usual pattern was to "take-off" with his two friends and some girls and go down to the park for the day to "get stoned." He indicated that he often would be on drugs for a month at a time, cutting classes at college during all that time. Heavy rock is his favorite kind of music; and he enjoyed music and reading prior to the accident. When questioned as to drugs *since* then, he first denied, then acknowledged, that he had been on marihuana about six times since then. He stated that he was through with them because the last time he had taken them, his speech and motor performance became much worse. As he recounted this, he laughed often, "It really must have been funny; wish I'd of had a tape recorder because of some of the funny things I said."

It would appear that the problems this young man was having prior to the accident are still very much a factor, even though he realizes in a vague sort of way that continued use of drugs or alcohol reduces his abilities even more.

SUMMARY: The right hemiparesis and resulting brain damage from the automobile accident have placed additional problems upon this client. It is unlikely that he would produce in a college setting, which is his goal at this time, due to factors of comprehension, memory, and the ability to recall language. The tenuous and difficult home situation adds to the already high level of anxiety of this patient.

RECOMMENDATIONS: Immediate counseling for alleviation of the depressed state, to be followed by vocational counseling and training in the direction of more realistic vocational goals.

Case #2 is unusual in that this twenty-two-year-old girl described had a very small section of her brain removed to save her life. Her adjustment to the resulting problems (especially in reading) is influenced favorably by her intelligence and education.

TESTS ADMINISTERED:
Wechsler Intelligence Scale
Wepman Aphasia Screening Test
Sensory Perceptual Examination
Tactual Performance Test
Halsted Category Test
Trailmaking Test
Figure Oscillation Test
Hand Dynamometer

DESCRIPTION OF SUBJECT: M. was seen as a part of a multidisciplinary evaluation two years after contracting meningeal encephalitis with subsequent neurosurgery in the left temporal area. Since that time she has been functionally alexic despite remedial reading and speech therapy.

M. was seen in interview before entering the testing situation. She related well and was cooperative and friendly. There was no noticeable communication difficulties, although on occasion M. appeared to become very confused when the conversation strayed from very direct and familiar areas. This confusion appeared to be present whether the task involved receptive or expressive ability on M.'s part. However, there were no noticeable signs of asphasic symptoms on casual examination.

TEST INTERPRETATION: On the Wechsler Adult Intelligence Scale, M. achieved verbal performance and Full Scale IQ's of 73, 93, and 80, respectively, placing her at the low end of the dull-normal adult range of functioning. Considering the patient's attained educational level as a college junior, these scores represent a significant decrement in cognitive functioning. As can be inferred from the variability of test scores, the verbal abilities appeared to be most markedly affected and may be down as much as forty to fifty points. The extreme split would call into question the integrity of the left cerebral hemisphere and would suggest unusual laterality of effect. The amount of time that had elapsed since onset of the illness would tend to argue against the probability of further improvement in the verbal intelligence areas. On tests of higher level problem-solving skills M. also showed mild impairment with category test score of 47, minimally delayed trail making scores, and some difficulty in understanding test directions. However, the subject showed good abilities when the task involved complex and simple motor activities. There appeared to be minimal impairment in these areas. However, in complex motor activities there was significant, but very mild, impairment of the right hand, particularly when used in conjunction with the left. This finding is contrary to patient's report of no motor difficulty. The difference found was relatively minimal and could be missed even when subject was engaged in tennis or piano playing. There appeared to be no noticeable memory deficit, particularly when the task involved spacially oriented memory, i.e. memory for figures.

In line with the WAIS scores the subject's most noticeable difficulties were apparent on the Halsted Wechsler Aphasia Screening Test and the Sensory Perceptual Examination. Although the subject appeared to have no difficulty in terms of constructional dyspraxia, she was unable to correctly identify or spell the words square, cross, and triangle. For example, she incorrectly identified the picture of a square as a circle. Considering the subject's level of alertness and her previous educational level, the performance was far below what one would expect. Since spacial difficulties did not appear to be involved, the effect seemed to be that of a significant dysnomia. Similarly the subject had significant difficulty in reading and dictation. She could however, copy simple words, i.e. square, when a model was provided. Arithmetic skills appeared to be less involved, but subject did experience some problems in this area. In addition there were minimal signs of right-left confusion. All signs are consistent with significant and static involvement of the left cerebral hemisphere, particularly in the temporal area with relative sparing of the right cerebral hemisphere.

On the Sensory Perceptual Examination subject showed no signs of difficulty in the tactile, auditory, or visual modalities under single or bilateral simultaneous stimulation. The finger agnosia subtest was also within normal limits as was the Fingertip Number Writing subtest. Subject appeared to have mild difficulty on the dysteragnosis subtest where stimulation involved correct identification of coins, particularly on the right side.

SUMMARY AND CONCLUSIONS: Test data are remarkably consistent in suggesting moderate, static, chronic lateralized impairment of the left cerebral hemisphere with consequent difficulties in verbal intelligence, language skills (whether expressive or receptive), and arithmetic areas. There appeared to be a very mild impairment of the right hand when complex motor activity was involved or when the task involved tactile identification of coins. In general, however, there was relative sparing of the sensory, perceptual, and simple motor areas.

In view of the subject's time past lesion and the amount of professional care which she has received it appears unlikely at this time that there will be a significant recovery of language functioning. Subject does, however, retain good skills in the performance areas and would appear to be employable if given the proper guidance in placement. Training and job activities should not involve a language area to any great extent although the subject is able to handle oral speech at a fairly reasonable level. The performance skills are good, and she relates well in interview and in general appears to be an excellent candidate for rehabilitation. She is now being considered for the residential program, and it would appear that this might be a good place for her on a cooperative basis with Vocational Rehabilitation and Easter Seal.

SUMMARY

Aphasia is the disruption of language in adults or the failure of langauge development in children due to damage to the part of the brain that controls language. Aphasia may vary greatly in severity and can involve the expression and/or the reception of language in its many forms. The chief specialist involved in the treatment and diagnosis of language disorders besides the physician is the speech therapist or speech pathologist. However, psychologists, audiologists, and social workers may be involved depending on the nature and complexity of the case. The duration and timing of therapy in cases of aphasia is critical to the speed and extent of recovery. The following agencies may be of benefit:

National
1. National Easter Seal
2. National Association of Hearing and Speech Agencies
Local
1. Speech Therapy

  a. college or university departments
  b. private or state agencies (see yellow pages)
2. Rehabilitation Centers
3. Easter Seal Society
4. Vocational Rehabilitaiton

Chapter 5

SEIZURES

General Definition

A SEIZURE is uncontrolled electrochemical activity in the brain usually producing movement effects and changes of consciousness. Recurrent seizures are labeled *epilepsy*. Since a variety of conditions can cause seizures, including fevers, tumors, and alcohol, seizures should be considered to be symptoms of an underlying process rather than a disease itself.

Voluntary movement is the end product of a complex biological chain: the brain through the nerve fibers to the voluntary muscles. Voluntary movements, including walking, talking, smiling, are all controlled by the appropriate electrochemical functioning of the brain. Uncontrolled electrochemical bursts in the brain produce the characteristic involuntary motor movements of seizures.

Any human being is capable of having a seizure. For most of us the body's resistance to a seizure is high enough so that we never experience one. If we do have a seizure, it is cause for alarm and anxiety. Seizures can be induced in normal individuals by high fevers (especially children); various drugs, including alcohol, in large quantities; and a variety of neurological conditions. The seizure is a sign or symptom of that condition. In such cases, the primary problem is to identify the underlying medical cause and eliminate it. Except in the rare case where seizures do not self-limit (stop) they are typically harmless to the body.

EPILEPSY

Despite the universal potential for seizures in all of us or perhaps because of it, few neurological conditions are regarded with more fear and misinformation. The person with recurrent

44

seizures, or epilepsy, is classified legally in some states with the insane and the feebleminded and is often barred unjustifiably from some jobs and activities. This rigidly negative attitude is changing, but too slowly.

An epileptic, for whatever medical reason, has a lowered physical threshold for recurrent seizures. Sometimes external precipitating conditions can be found that trigger the seizures. The conditions may be as commonplace as flickering fluorescent bulbs, sunlight along a tree-shaded highway, or simple fatigue. Where an external precipitating cause is known, some success has been achieved in desensitizing the individual to the cause. The process is not too dissimilar to getting accustomed to allergy-producing objects by gradually increasing exposure to the objects (desensitization). Where desensitization is not possible, avoidance of the seizure producing conditions is necessary. Unfortunately, usually there is no triggering condition that can be observed. The individual has recurrent seizures without warning or apparent cause.

Medical Control

In 80 percent of the cases, good control of the seizures can be accomplished with medication. Strict adherence to the medical regiment can allow the individual a normal and productive life.

Behavioral Effects

Unlike many neurological conditions, recurrent seizures do not necessarily imply any specifiable personality or cognitive difficulties. If the seizures are caused by a demonstrable condition, i.e. a tumor or head injury, then indeed, personality and cognitive changes may be associated in the individual case. Seizures by themselves do not reflect behavioral abnormalities.

By contrast, much has been written about the *epileptic personality*. Typically, these statements are based on comparison studies in which a group of seizure-prone individuals are given some standard personality or intelligence test and compared to the normal population. When the medical group varies in some way (usually negatively) from the general group, the implication is made that

1. All seizure-prone individuals display these negative characteristics.
2. The differences found occur all the time.
3. The differences are caused by the same brain abnormalities that cause the seizures.

The truth is we really do not know for certain whether epilepsy always causes negative and invariable behavioral shifts. Considering the wide diversity of conditions that can cause seizures and the wide range of individual variability, such consistency of bad effects seems at best improbable. Poor adjustment may go along with a seizure disorder, but the effect should be considered neither uniform nor universal.

However, consider for a moment how it would be to be an epileptic, to be barred from certain activities and professions, to have a condition that other people regard as disturbing or even somehow sinful, to never quite know whether without warning your body may fail you and abruptly propel you into a helpless and possibly endangered state. Under that kind of stress, the most stable individual might become somewhat suspicious and negative toward the attitudes and behaviors of other people, not quite certain of those around them.

In summary, perhaps if there are differences in the behavior of people who have seizures it may be largely because people treat them differently and expect differences from them. We sometimes get what we expect from people.

Genetic Factors

There are many possible causes for seizures. A few of them are genetic and as such can be transmitted as an inherited predisposition to later generations. The ethics and the probabilities of such a predisposition are a matter of medical advice and individual conscience. If epilepsy in a given individual is inherited and transmittable, then the individual owes it to his spouse and to his future children to learn as much as he can about the condition and its probabilities. Your physician can advise you or refer you to another source of information.

Types of Seizures

There are four major types of seizures — major motor, petit mal, Jacksonian, and psychomotor. Each has a characteristic pattern which may or may not resemble the stereotyped view of a *fit*. Some seizures are so minimal in duration and external behavioral changes that people around the individual may not recognize the seizure. Often an individual will have more than one type. However, even when the disturbing external signs of the condition are not blatant, the individual still suffers at least some alteration of consciousness during the time of the seizure. His relative alertness and efficiency may therefore be influenced without his awareness.

Major Motor

Major motor seizures are those with highly visible characteristics disturbing to the individual and to his family. As with most seizure disorders, however, this condition can often be controlled with medication.

Major motor seizures may be preceded by warning feelings (auras) experienced by the patient, such as flashing lights, strange sounds, or peculiar smells or feelings, such as anxiety. The type of aura may be related to the part of the brain prone to electrochemical imbalance. The individual is not really exposed to these sensory stimuli but perceives them as sensory warning that his brain is about to go into the extreme electrochemical imbalance that is the internal manifestation of the seizure.

Characteristically, an individual having a Major motor seizure falls to the ground with an exhaled cry. There are three sources of danger to the individual that are described — physical damage from the fall, biting the tongue during the seizure, or swallowing the tongue. Simple precautions can usually prevent the first two problems. Your physician will be happy to go over these procedures with you. The folklore of "swallowing the tongue" would quickly vanish if those repeating the danger would try to swallow their own tongues. What seems to be a swallowed tongue is the air passing over the relaxed tongue of the individual and creating a disturbing rattle. Turn the individual to the side and it disappears. Three stages follow the beginning of the major motor seizure:

1. *Tonic* stage in which the body maintains a stiff, rigid posture.

2. *Clonic* stage in which alternating muscle spasms produce the characteristic spasms. Bowel and bladder control may be lost.

3. A period of unconsciousness/stupor may follow.

A fairly rare and dangerous state occurs if the individual has one seizure after another. Seizures are usually self-limiting, i.e. stop themselves. If seizures do not self-limit, the patient is in a genuine medical emergency, and a physician *must* be summoned.

Petit Mal

Petit mal seizures may be so minimal in behavioral effects that a child may have several seizures a day without anyone being aware. The effects can be so slight that even a trained observer may miss them. Muscle responses may be as minimal as slight facial twitching or rapid eye blinking for a few seconds.

Petit mal seizures typically involve a brief period of loss of awareness without periods of confusion or gross motor effects. The individual may abruptly interrupt his speech, stare, and then go on without awareness of any gap in consciousness or time. The only definitive way to determine the presence of petit mal seizures is by the specialized medical technique of the electro-encephalogram (EEG).

A child with unsuspected seizures may appear to daydream or to be inattentive. Certainly, if as often happens, the attacks appear in clusters, or showers, of up to several hundred a day, the individual may have a significant learning handicap. The child who unknowingly flickers in and out of consciousness will miss much of what the teacher is saying or doing. Since the first step in learning has to involve some visual or auditory cue which the person perceives and acts on, the first step of the learning chain may be interrupted frequently. Even a bright child has a substantial disadvantage to overcome such conditions. The child cannot remember what he did not perceive. Proper diagnosis and medical control can have definitely positive effects.

Jacksonian

Jacksonian seizures begin in one part of the body, often an arm or a leg, and spread in area and intensity throughout the body. They are said to *march* from the effected site. Like the characteristic aura that may accompany seizures, the part of the body that begins to seizure is a clue to the part of the brain that is affected.

Psychomotor

Psychomotor seizures are puzzling variants on the usual picture of uncontrolled muscle activity. An individual having a psychomotor seizure may carry out complicated activities without memory. At the time, the patient may appear to be in a trance, may fly into an uncontrolled rage, or otherwise demonstrate an abrupt unexplainable behavioral shift bordering on the bizarre. Truly dangerous or destructive acts are rare. Memory loss or partial memory loss are usual. The auras associated with such seizures, when they occur, are also highly variable, including changes in perception of time or distance, sounds, and the deja vu experience of feeling something has happened before.

Diagnosis

The most common method of diagnosing seizures is through use of the elctroencehpalogram (EEG). Despite its imposing name and highly complicated appearance, the procedure is completely safe. Basically, the EEG does nothing more than pick up, from several electrodes placed on the scalp, the electrical activity of the brain, much like a radio receiver picks up the radio signals in the air. The machine itself does nothing to the individual. It is a completely passive procedure. The electrical activity of the brain is translated into movements of a pen over a moving paper tape. The tape record is read by a physician specially trained in the area. The major side effect to the patient is the somewhat messy globs of electrode paste that have to be washed out of the hair.

CASE STUDY

The following case illustrates three important points discussed in the text of the chapter.

1. Seizures are only one symptom of an underlying condition which may have other unsuspected effects.

2. Learning problems associated with brain damage may produce behavior difficulties in the young through frustration.

3. Re-evaluations (medical or others) are often necessary in the young patient because of the unreliability of any testing in the very young and because children change as they grow.

TESTS ADMINISTERED: Three Performance subtests of the Wechsler Intelligence Scale for Children (WISC): Picture Completion, Block Design, and Object Assembly.

Halstead-Category Test
Matching Pictures Test
Individual Performance Tests:
    Matching V's, Star, Matching Figures, Concentric
    Squares
Finger Tapping Speed
Strength of Grip (Dynamometer)
Tests of Dominance
Children's Form of Wepman-Halstead Aphasia Screening Test
Goodenough-Harris Draw-A-Woman

PRESENTING PROBLEM: This child was referred to the clinic of the center for a complete speech evaluation as well as some indications of psychological and intellectual functioning. R. has a medical history indicating epileptic seizures from the age of six months and continuing periodically. She was seen for a speech evaluation and subsequently received three months of speech therapy. Since placement in a regular first grade classroom in the public schools, this child appears to be unable to cope with the usual learning tasks, whimpers and cries if frustrated, and often refuses to respond.

PREVIOUS TESTING PERFORMED: A Peabody Picture Vocabulary Test given 2-26 indicated an M.A. of two to eight years. Readministration of the PPVT showed a growth in M.A. of two years. Several tests of visual perception, manual dexterity, and gross motor development indicated R. was functioning at about the four to four and one-half year level. Speech and language evaluation could not be completed due to the behavior of the child. A hearing screening completed at this time indicated hearing within normal limits.

OBSERVATIONS OF BEHAVIOR: R. appeared reluctant to go with the examiner and would only do so when her mother accompanied her to the testing room. The examiner relied upon the newness and uniqueness of the testing apparatus in the room to interest her, rather than attempting to verbalize with her. The Halstead Category Test was begun immediately, and the pictures on the screen and colored lights appeared to lessen the child's apprehensiveness. The examiner felt that it was only because so little verbalization was demanded of R. that she cooperated as much as she did. Her trembling and "about-to-cry" expression soon diminished, and R. attempted almost all of the tests presented to her. She was told at the beginning of the session that she could have a jelly bean from a jar after the completion of each test, and she enjoyed getting these and counting them (incorrectly).

R. became very upset whenever a test demanded a speech response, no matter how minimal. She could only sustain this type of testing for a very short time. The examiner could anticipate her increase in apprehensiveness by her increased swallowing, trembling lower lip, and latent responses. By switching to another test she could be sustained for longer periods of time.

R. flatly refused to take the astereognosis and Fingertip Writing sections of the Aphasia Screening. These tests required that she put her hand through a foam rubber gasket mounted on a standing board. No amount of explaining or demonstration on the part of the examiner could convince her that there was nothing on the other side that could possibly hurt her. She also became fearful when she discovered that the Tactual Performance Test required that she had to be blindfolded. When the examiner let R. place the blindfold on her, the child agreed to take the test. She performed for only about fifteen to thirty seconds. The combination of the blindfold and the difficult task of placing the blocks on the board apparently were too much for her. She began to cry and removed the blindfold. This reaction appears to be fairly typical of the behavior that may be expected when R. is faced with a new and unfamiliar situation. It would be important to consider for any therapeutic approaches.

Constant reassurance and a great deal of praise were necessary on the part of the examiner to sustain R. throughout the three-hour testing period.

INTERPRETATION: The very poor level of functioning on the performance subtests of the WISC may be indicative of very little spatial ability and present evidence of organicity.

Poor concept formation abilities were observed in the overall performance on the Halstead Category Test. As soon as the first subtest was completed (score: 9 out of 10), R. began to have difficulty when the more abstract concepts of similarities and differences were presented.

The low level of concept formation was substantiated by the showing on the Matching Pictures Test, where increasingly more difficult levels of generalization must be applied. Only the simplest parts of this test battery were completed with any success.

The four tests which comprise the Individual Performance Test Battery suggested a limited level of expressive and receptive aspects of visuo-spatial relationships have been developed. Close attention to design and detail are necessary. R. performed poorly, as shown not only by the few points scored correctly, but also by the amount of time taken to complete the tasks.

Finger Tapping Speed and Strength of Grip were within normal limits. R. showed a tendency to use both right hand and right foot for most tasks. The few times she used her left hand and foot do not comprise enough evidence to support an indication of confusion of laterality.

Gross sensory-perceptual functioning (tactile, visual, auditory) was normal. As noted previously, the more sophisticated tests of this part of the Aphasia Screening were not completed. R. was reluctant to do any tests which necessitated lengthy directions or unusual tasks. Observation of her drawings indicated deterioration with each repetition of the drawing; with the Greek Cross being especially poor. She was unable to read and could copy the arithmetic problem 2 + 1, but could not solve it; nor could she verbally solve the problem 2 + 2.

The Goodenough-Harris drawing placed R. in the lowest percentile and suggested an IQ of about 60.

SUMMARY COMMENTS: This seven and one-half year old child appears apprehensive and fearful of situations and tasks involving higher level functioning, particularly those involving verbalization, spatial concepts, abstraction, and formation of concept learning. She is approximately three years behind in terms of cognitive learning tasks. Right-left body comparisons appear within normal limits. Gross functioning in sensory-perceptual areas is normal; more discrete testing could not be accomplished.

In view of the findings of the tests in this battery, it is understandable that R. is finding it increasingly difficult to function in the normal classroom situation. Her limited speech production prevents her from adequate communication, and her depressed intelligence makes her rely upon the understanding and support of those in her immediate environment. It is doubtful that she has ever been placed in a searching, exploring situation for learning that was controlled and reduced to her level.

Cerebral dysfunction appears to be diffuse, involving both hemispheres. Some emotional overlay also appears to be operating. There is a discrepancy in the behavioral observations of this child two years ago and those which the staff have observed. Her outgoing attitude, cooperativeness, and affectionate behavior now have been replaced by a fearfulness and withdrawal from new and threatening situations.

RECOMMENDATIONS: It is recommended that R. be withdrawn from the regular classroom situation and be placed in a special education class, if such a placement is possible.

Speech and language therapy is also suggested. Behavior modification techniques may prove to be effective with R., beginning at the level of immediate reward for any verbalization.

Re-examination by a neurologist and EEG's. The last EEG's were apparently completed when this child was quite young, as evidenced by the records available.

SUMMARY

Seizures may be caused by many conditions. They usually can be controlled by medication once the underlying causes are treated. They are not typically dangerous themselves. Seizures do not necessarily cause behavioral or emotional disturbances. When an individual does have seizures, however, he must

1. Maintain close contact with his physician, including regular medical checkups.

2. Take his medication.

3. Avoid, when possible, conditions that can lower his seizure threshold, i.e. alcohol, fatigue, emotional stress, or drugs.

4. Be aware if the condition underlying his seizures may be inherited.

5. Be given immediate medical care if his seizures start and do not stop.

6. Check with his physician regarding limitations on potentially dangerous activities such as driving.

Chapter 6

CEREBRAL PALSY

GENERAL DEFINITION

CEREBRAL palsy (CP) is an inability to control voluntary muscle movement because of damage to the brain. Any voluntary movement requires

1. Simple movement of the primary muscle.

2. Smooth coordination of the primary muscle with another muscle or set of muscles acting in the opposite direction to dampen or control the movement.

3. Finely timed transfer of the simple movement to the next movement when the act requires a chain or sequence of motions, i.e. picking up a glass is not one movement of a single muscle but a series of many movements and muscles.

4. Precise control of the force, extent, and direction of the movement.

5. Stopping the movement at the proper time. Damage to any or all of these steps can produce the characteristic movements of CP.

Severity of the effect can vary from mild to sufficiently severe so as to require extensive medical and/or rehabilitation efforts. Although CP can be inherited, it is far more usual that some other cause, i.e. birth trauma, anoxia, or head injuries, have so damaged the brain so as to make voluntary movement uncoordinated and difficult.

Cerebral palsy is really not a single disease, but a whole host of nonprogressive conditions loosely classified together because motor effects are one of the more visible features. The two most common types of muscle control problems are called spastic cerebral palsy and athetoid cerebral palsy. Spacicity refers to uncontrolled, unselective overtightness of muscles. For movement to occur, the muscles opposite to the muscles contracting should be relatively relaxed. When they are not, the movement is spastic. Athetoid movement disorders involve an inability to stop a single movement once begun. The effect of athetoid involvement is to produce a *wormlike* exaggerated movement. The cause of the condition (which is static, i.e. never getting worse once it occurs) can range from a lack of oxygen at birth to some small cell defect in the brain. Unfortunately, the term cerebral palsy is so emotionally loaded that people react to the term rather than the particular characteristics of the person.

SEIZURES

Seizures may occur with cerebral palsy since both are caused by damage to the central nervous system (see Ch. 5). The diagnosis and treatment of seizures is medical and requires a close cooperative relationship between the patient and his physician. In the great majority of cases, medication can be of great benefit to the patient.

LANGUAGE EFFECTS

Speech involves many muscles in its productions: lips, tongue, breathing, soft palate, etc. These muscles must operate together in the proper sequence and at the proper rate. If muscle movement is not coordinated, articulation problems may occur and the individual's speech may be unintelligible even in context. In addition, reception, integration, and expression of language is mediated by the brain, especially the left hemisphere of the brain. Because of the necessary interaction of voluntary muscle control, language usage, and the integrity of the brain, inarticulate or even unintelligible speech often accompanies cerebral palsy. If it does appear that an individual with CP has a speech problem, he should be evaluated by a speech therapist or speech pathologist as soon as practical. An early evaluation is important for two reasons.

1. The extent of the difficulty and whether it involves receptive, expressive, or just articulation problems can have important implications for future educational and vocational

planning (see chapter on aphasia).

2. The earlier that effective treatment can be initiated after diagnosis, the better for the individual from an emotional and educational standpoint.

INTELLIGENCE

The most common referral question to clinical psychologists involves the determination of intelligence, whether the question is being asked by parents, teachers, or physicians. Typically the person who refers the patient is concerned about learning ability in a traditional school setting. The parents of a youngster with cerebral palsy seeing the outward physical manifestations of the condition are usually anxious, whether they ask the specific question or not, to know if mental limitations are also part of the total picture. Is this child retarded?

Historically, intelligence tests were developed to give some objective way of picking out children with learning problems before they failed in a school system. Since school material is heavily verbal in nature, the usual intelligence tests are highly dependent on learned verbal skills, whether they are given individually or in groups.

Group Tests

Group intelligence tests, those usually given in a school setting, are helpful screening devices. Large numbers of individuals can be tested at one time and objective, easily scored results can assist in planning for placement, further testing, or counseling.

However, low scores, especially those generated on a group basis, may be a function of many variables. Anxiety, emotional disturbance, brain damage, cultural differences, and general health can all adversely effect test scores. An intelligence score is just that, a score on a test, and is not an unvarying number determined by direct physical examination. The individual being tested is usually asked to understand the verbal directions given to the class by the examiner, to relate those directions to the problems on the paper in front of him, and to work on his own until told to stop. Speed of response is important to the final score. An individual with cerebral palsy, if only because he cannot respond as rapidly as other individuals, is at considerable disadvantage in the group testing setting. For that reason, if intelligence is an issue in CP, the person should be given an individually administered intelligence test by a qualified examiner.

Individual Intelligence Tests

Individually administered tests are typically given by a psychologist (school or clinical) on a one-to-one basis over a time period of one hour or more. Sometimes it may be necessary to spread testing over two or more testing sessions if special problems in testing are encountered.

Intelligence tests given individually typically have both verbal and nonverbal items. Sometimes separate scores for verbal and nonverbal performance are computed to compare the individual scores with others in these tests at his age level. Depending on the severity of the motor involvement in the individual case, it is to be anticipated that individuals with cerebral palsy will not do as well as the general population on tasks requiring fine motor control, rapid eye-hand coordination, and manipulation of materials.

Verbal items more closely approximating school tasks may also be lower than the general population. There can be a number of explanations for such low scores.

1. The scores may reflect real cognitive limitations. Cerebral palsy implies some kind of brain damage which may lead to lowered abilities. In children, the most usual effect of brain damage is a lowering of intelligence as measured by group and individual tests.

2. Verbal answers must be scoreable. If speech problems are present, the individual's replies may be so garbled so as to not allow full credit. Often, an examiner may be concerned about not creating anxiety in the patient and may hesitate to ask the

individual to constantly repeat his answer beyond a reasonable limit.

3. The person being tested may have been so shielded from the environment by his family that he never accumulates the usual fund of knowledge and experience that most individuals acquire. Since intelligence test scores are somewhat dependent on early experience and learning, performance may be correspondingly lowered in an individual who has never been exposed to the usual amount of environmental stimulation. The child who has never attempted to solve a common puzzle on his own or who has never been asked to define a word can be expected to do poorly in such a task. The shielding of a handicapped individual by his family from whatever learning experiences may be available to him is neither kind nor helpful.

4. Finally, it should be remembered that intelligence test scores, like any other test dependent on a sample of performance at one given moment in time, may be lowered by a variety of situational or personal variables including anxiety, emotional disturbance, general health and motivation, and sensory loss (the hard of hearing youngster, for example). The examiner should have some idea of the validity of his testing and any probable contaminating factors.

PERSONALITY VARIABLES

A great deal of professional time and energy has been devoted to the description of the CP personality. Individuals with CP have been described as suspicious, aloof, emotionally volatile, naive, unstable, overly concerned with health matters, and hostile. Such a description or set of descriptive phrases seems more authoritative than it is and implies two things.

1. Every individual with CP, regardless of age, intelligence, degree of involvement, environment, underlying cause of the condition, and level of educational and vocational progress, will invariably act that way under most conditions.

2. The individual acts the way he does because his condition directly causes him to act that way, i.e. damage to the brain causes both the CP and the observed personality variables.

The first assumption is obviously unlikely. Cerebral palsy is a complex symptom extremely variable in its cause and effects imposed on an even more complex system (the human body and nervous system). It is unlikely that the effects of CP on personality are less complicated and more invariable than the physical effects.

The second assumption is more complicated than it first appears. An individual with CP has a condition which limits his ability to act or behave the way most people behave. Depending on the degree of involvement, many of the differences may be immediately visible to people in the environment. Typically speaking, an individual with a visible handicap will

1. be treated differently than others,

2. will be thought of in a different fashion than most people,

3. will be initially considered less able to deal with the demands of the environment regardless of the situation.

Briefly then, an individual with obvious CP will often be considered by those around him to be different. He need not interact or even speak in order to create a negative first impression; he is different on sight. The individual with cerebral palsy is considered first to have cerebral palsy and then to be an individual. Under such environmental conditions it would not be surprising to find personality characteristics shaped or molded into suppressiveness and hostility.

In a more subtle fashion and with the best of feelings and intentions, the family of the individual with cerebral palsy can do him a great disservice by shielding him. It is a truism in rehabilitation that "many are kind but few are helpful." Most of the learning processes and the acquisition of necessary social and intellectual skills depend on the opportunity to make mistakes. The baby cannot learn to walk without falling down; the ball player misses much more than he hits in the beginning. Learning always involves environmental opportunity. Without exposure to the learning situation and the chance to do poorly for a while, the individual cannot improve his performance. When someone in the family has a handicap, especially a child, it is difficult to avoid doing too much for him in meeting his physical needs and keeping him from being embarrassed or making mistakes in a social context. It is no favor to force a handicapped individual into dependence and to deny him the opportunity to develop the coping skills that he will neeed more than most people.

The line between independence and necessary dependence is a difficult line to draw. How far can the family go in promoting independence without endangering the physical or emotional health of the individual? That question is not one easily answered in general; it can only be tentatively attempted in a specific case at a specific time. The handicapped child or adult is a person first and has a handicap second. They always deserve the benefit of doubt; they always deserve the opportunity to make choices appropriate to their age, and they always deserve the opportunity that the rest of us enjoy — to be absolutely, completely, and without reservation, inept.

CASE STUDY

The following case (which includes two reports) illustrates the adjustment problems of a young man who acquired motor control problems through an accident. He is married, has children, and until the time of the accident had been a highly skilled worker. The patient's adjustment to his new limitations is a good one.

TESTS ADMINISTERED:
Sensory-Perceptual Secton of Wepman-Halstead Aphasia
    Screening Test
Speed of Finger Tapping
Strength of Grip (Dynamometer)
Tactual Performance Test

OBSERVATION OF BEHAVIOR: The examiner was immediately impressed with the social awareness skills and ease with which the client entered into the testing situation. His command of the language was explicit and direct, but in terms of clinical impressions this ease and skill rapidly deteriorated when O. became at all frustrated or upset.

Articulation was dysarthric, characterized by slurring of consonant bldnds and imprecise production of consonants. During the course of this brief battery of tests, speech production would become worse if the situation upset or frustrated the client.

O. was cooperative and more than willing to discuss his developmental history. He mentioned that he was not really sure whether or not he had polio. His mother had told him that he did not start to walk until he was over two years of age. He states that he has always been bothered by a weakness and numbness in his right side. If he runs, the numbness will begin in his right hand and travel up the arm and shoulder to the right side of his head. He now uses his left hand for most tasks where fine movement or strength is required.

INTERPRETATION: There is an apparent right-left determination problem which may contribute to O.'s slowness in performing motoric tasks. Finger Tapping was quite labored with both hands, but was in the direction to be expected from hand preference. Grip strength is less for the right hand, but is within normal limits if the left hand is now dominant, as the client states.

During the Tactual Performance Test with the left hand, mild athetotic movements of the right fingers and the head and neck were noted. O. had to rest three times, and finally stated that he was dizzy and wanted to stop. The performance time is very slow.

Fingertip Number Writing produced many errors. There may have been several factors operating: (1) the build-up in frustration level from the previous tasks; (2) it could not be clearly determined beforehand whether or not O. can readily recognize the numbers; and (3) the fact that the numbers are written upside-down may have been too difficult for him.

There was difficulty in tactile recognition of the coins used, and some astereognosis appeared to be present.

CONCLUSIONS: There is evidence from these tests that some CNS damage has occurred, primarily to the left hemisphere. Some diffuse damage may also be present in the right hemisphere. Situations of stress are not handled well, and fine motor tasks produce frustration and increase the symptoms noted above under OBSERVATION OF BEHAVIOR. Further organic testing does not appear to be necessary, since substantial evidence of organic impairment has already been noted. It might be reasonable to consider that his reading problem may be accounted for in part by this left hemisphere involvement.

This may be a consideration in terms of prognosis.

Report II — Same Individual

O. is a twenty-seven-year-old male who has been diagnosed as a victim of cerebral palsy. As a result of this condition, he experiences pain in his arms and legs and has some difficulties with motor coordination and speech. He is currently employed as a laborer. He and his wife, who is unemployed, have small children. His interests include hunting, building, and drawing.

In terms of physical appearance, he is a rather good-looking man whose athetoid movements are only moderately noticeable. He was dressed neatly for the testing session and seemed to have no trouble interacting with the examiner. He took the testing quite seriously and evidenced anxiety and frustration on several occasions.

O.'s greatest periods of anxiety were marked by a deterioration in speech.

On the WAIS, he obtained a Verbal Scale IQ of 89 and a Performance Scale IQ of 84, for a Full Scale score of 86. This placed him in the dull-normal range of intellectual functioning. A WAIS administered in 1963 also revealed achievement within this range.

In terms of verbal ability, the client is average with respect to skills involving social judgment and abstraction. His below average performance of subscales reflecting knowledge of information, vocabulary, and arithmetic probably reflect his lack of education and poor development of academic skills (e.g. WRAT reading=grade 2.4; spelling=grade 2.2; arithmetic=grade 2.3). His immediate memory ability is also below par, but this was possibly a reflection of anxiety. Scores on performance items reflect his poor motor coordination. There do seem to be indications of an ability to plan and to synthesize visual materials, not surprising considering the patient's background.

In the way of personality functioning, O. is very conscious of his disability and appears rather distressed by it. In an attempt to compensate, he has become very achievement oriented and expresses a great need to demonstrate independence in his activities. His history and this testing session reveal an individual who tries very hard, becomes frustrated at times, but seems to manage to pick himself up and try again.

SUMMARY AND RECOMMENDATIONS: O. is a twenty-seven-year-old male who exhibits intellectual functioning within the dull-normal range. His high motivation and his average abilities in the way of judgment, abstraction, and planning appear to make him suitable for training. He is limited by his inability to read and spell, though he would probably respond well to instruction in these areas. His physical disability will limit vocational choice: motor coordination, particularly fine motor skills, is limited and physical labor, in which he is currently engaged, is difficult and painful.

SUMMARY AND RECOMMENDATIONS

Cerebral palsy is a group of nonprogressive disorders characterized by lack of muscle control. A variety of causes can produce CP, and the effects can vary from mild to severe and may involve

1. Seizures
2. Speech, language, and articulation difficulties
3. Limitations in learning ability

Once the diagnosis of CP has been made medically, the family should consider the following steps:

1. Physical Therapy and Occupational Therapy evaluations to assist in the physical restoration and prevention (see final chapter).
2. Speech evaluation if language or articulation lags developmentally.
3. Psychological evaluation when the child is three or older to assist in school planning.
4. Early contact with the school system for knowledge of special classes that may be available.
5. Contact the national and local branch of the United Cerebral Palsy Association.

Chapter 7

AGING

THE average age of the population of the United States is increasing. The combination of a dropping birthrate and advances in medical care have produced a larger and larger segment of our population beyond the age of fifty. With increasing numbers of old people, there has naturally evolved a greater and greater incidence of medical, personal, and social problems associated with the aging process.

Unfortunately, the sociological changes that occur at the same time have created more problems for the aged. Families are smaller, more mobile, and less close. There is no longer room or the expectation for caring for someone past retirement age. In consequence, growing old for many people has meant poverty or even institutionalization. Many of those in mental hospitals are not insane, but are simply old and have no place to go.

Increases in social security and the medicare program suggest that old people are rediscovering their franchise. Economic and medical difficulties, while still major problems, are at least being studied and considered. However, the emotional and mental aspects of the aging, to date, are still relatively ignored or clouded by tradition. Adequate medical care and financial support are basic necessities for a dignified existence, old or young, but they are only a part of the picture. Each man must come to terms with himself and with his environment when he can no longer work and when his thinking processes are altered by age. This is a developmental task at least as important and difficult as adolescence.

ADJUSTMENT OF AGING AS A DEVELOPMENTAL TASK

There is a decade from thirty-five to forty in many individuals' lives characterized by depression and emotional upheaval. It has been suggested that this period marks the transition zone into awareness of increasing age. Certainly at this time physical decline begins to make itself felt.

The gradual decline of physical abilities and the far more slow and subtle lowering of mental agility culminates eventually in retirement and death. According to folklore and the insurance industry, the final period of a man's life is the *golden years.* Without adequate preparation, the golden years can be a time of frustration, disillusionment, and emotional decline.

For good or bad, many of us identify our feeling of personal worth with our work. When our usual way of spending our time and proving ourselves is taken away, even temporarily as on a long vacation, we feel edgy and bored. If a person is forced by age to retire, he is cut loose from the activities that filled his time and gave it meaning. An individual who has been totally job oriented and who has not developed his leisure time interests will probably attempt to cling to powers and achievements of the past. Such a defense mechanism is understandable but difficult to accept for those around the aged person: his wife (who has him underfoot); his children (who are at the full peak of their abilities); his peers (who may or may not still be alive). No wonder, then, with decreased mobility, lowered spending power, increased time, and T.V., the old person begins to be described as touchy, living in the past, and lacking in mental acuity. With the rapid shifts in society, the older person who does not keep himself informed and involved becomes increasingly dislocated in time as well as in ability from those around him.

MENTAL SHIFTS IN AGING

Three points must be made before discussing the usual effects of aging.

1. There is extreme variability from individual to individual in the impact of aging on mental facility. Some people are grossly affected before their sixtieth birthday. Others are alert and able beyond ninety. The effects to be noted later are generalities of varying significance in the particular case.

2. There appears to be good evidence that the individual who stays interested and involved in his environment beyond the point

of planning for his future career is much more likely to stay alert and mentally sharp.

3. There are not yet recognized medical treatments to slow or reverse the effects of aging on the brain. There is, however, much research going on in this area, especially as it pertains to blood vessel diseases. Vast promises as to expensive cures for aging with vitamins, pills, and other treatments should be taken with a grain of salt.

Structurally, there are many changes that happen with aging. The brain loses weight; the grooves that divide the brain widen and deepen. Probably most fundamental to the mental changes is the decreasing ability of the body to supply adequate amounts of blood (and therefore oxygen to the brain cells. The brain requires more oxygen than any other organ. Without adequate amounts of oxygen, the brain cannot operate at peak efficincy.

VERBAL ABILITY CHANGES

Verbal abilities, as measured by typical intelligence testing, are retained better than most other skills. The older person may be described as overtalkative and garrulous when in fact he is capitalizing on his greatest remaining strength and de-emphasizing the areas of weakness. Three major points are important here.

1. Verbal skills are typically old stored material and as such do not represent the need for verbal problem solving. Those skills may be more impaired.

2. The older person's relatively intact verbal skills can mask real impairment. For example, an individual may be able to achieve a superior intelligence test score and "sound good" and be unable to handle emergency situations when they arise.

3. It is essential that the older individual continue to take in, via verbal channels, new material and information about the world. The verbal channel is often the most intact ability left to the older individual and must be used to allow him to cope and shift with the outside world. For that reason, adult education, reading, and mass media (regretably to a lesser extent) are not only useful but perhaps essential to the continued development of the

person as other sources and channels are reduced or stopped.

PERFORMANCE SKILLS

It is axiomatic that we "slow down" with aging. Reflexes, muscle strength, sensory acuity, are all subject to deterioration and change from the peak period in the early twenties. However, as inevitable as these changes are, several strategies of coping can be helpful.

1. Transportation can often be a problem. The individual should consider the possibility of annual re-examination in driving skills, even if his state does not require it, for his safety and that of others. He should further consider availability of public transportation or extremely close goods and service facilities.

2. A regular exercise program began early can slow physical deterioration and reduce the probability of health and reasoning endangering conditions, e.g. strokes.

3. Regular medical checkups are vital since the old no longer have the health reserves to fight off minor problems.

4. Nutrition in the old is often neglected. Appetite, income, and taste often deteriorate and can lead to a protein and vitamin deficient diet.

NEW LEARNING

There is little question that one's ability to learn new material is reduced with aging. Studies have consistently indicated that the complexity of the material, the length of time available for learning, and the amount of rapid problem solving necessary are all key variables for the older person. In general, the more complex, the more extensive, the shorter the time span, and the greater the amount of decision making required by the task, the more deficient an older individual will look.

However, it should be emphasized that the same studies which pointed up areas of difficulty also found one key point: *The ability to learn is not destroyed by the normal aging process. Given sufficient time and assuming material within the reasoning abilities of the older person, the older individual can and should continue to learn throughout his life.*

MEMORY PROBLEMS

Memory difficulties are commonly associated with the aging process. Typically, memory deficiencies are those of new learning rather than past experiences. The older individual can sometimes remember with astonishing clarity what happened when he was thirty, but may forget from one hour to the next the name of someone he has just met.

Memory difficulties may involve any of three separate processes or combinations:

1. Immediate or short-term memory: The individual cannot register the information to be remembered even on a short-term basis. He may forget within moments the date to be remembered.

2. Problems in the short-term to long-term memory shift: It is recognized that different processes and probably different neural patterns are required in short-term and long-term memory and that physiological processes linking the two can break down. What this means to the individual can be a relatively intact short-term memory (a few hours in duration), but an inability to retain over longer periods.

3. Retrieval difficulties may exist: If a memory is regarded as a bit of information in storage, the individual may have difficulty in locating and expressing the precise memory or word needed; it may be "right on the tip of his tongue." It is as if the brain's filing system were faulty, and bits and pieces of information were piled in untidy heaps.

Suggestions for Memory Difficulties

Memory difficulties have been measured and studied extensively. What to do about memory problems from aging is far less adequately handled. However, the following procedures may assist the individual.

1. Mnemonic devices: See any of the popular books and articles on memory enhancement, such as October, 1973, issue of *Psychology Today.*

2. Systematizing and structuring procedures: It is sometimes helpful for the individual to become more involved and systematic in the memory process and utilize preplanning, scheduling, outlining, and review procedures to organize material to be learned.

3. Artificial aids such as notebooks, lists, and set routines while cumbersome can, in part, support and reinforce the memory process.

4. Overlearning, i.e. more study and repetitions of new material may be necessary.

ABNORMAL AGING PROCESSES

The aging process is a natural function of living, and the changes associated with it, though requiring major adjustments, are usually sufficiently gradual so as to allow dignity and alertness to the end. However, with some individuals, and especially now as more and more people live beyond the sixties, there are severe mental changes associated with aging.

Senile Psychosis

In any person who ages, certain physical changes occur to the brain. The blood flow is diminished, the brain loses weight, changes occur in the cells and arteries. As with every physical, emotional, and mental attribute of man, there is enormous variation in the rapidity and the severity of these physical changes and of the associated symptoms. When the mental changes are sufficient so as not to allow the individual contact with the external world and when he can no longer be trusted to live independently, a senile psychosis can be said to occur.

Typically, the onset of senility is gradual and may represent an overaccentuation of a preexisting trait. The hostile or suspicious person may become more so. Confusion, suspiciousness, emotional difficulty, and depression may all be part of the clinical picture. Suicide and depression may occur. A physical can advise and help with medication and dietary supplements, but severe brain damage from aging is usually considered as irreversible and progressive. Medical science is exploring many avenues including drugs, hyperbaric chambers, and other experimental techniques, but to date there are no real answers.

If psychosis has developed, institutionalization must be considered, probably as a terminal placement. Your physician may advise you as to placement and financial possibilities. Consider other alternatives to hospitalization. Twenty to 25 percent of the patients in public mental hospitals are the aged. However, the lack of funds in many state institutions may allow no more than caretaking facilities. Consider asking for assistance from a social work agency, i.e. county health department of university department of social welfare, in the selection and financing areas.

Rare Aging Processes

Some rare conditions, specifically Picks and Alzheimer's disease, represent accelerated aging processes of unknown cause. Because disease processes occur so rapidly and completely, it is usual that public care is the only alternative, since the patient is so debilitated as to be considered psychotic.

RECOMMENDATIONS IN SUMMARY FORM

For clarity the following suggestions are made in list form.

1. See a physician routinely and report immediately any sudden physical, behavioral, emotional, or reasoning shifts to him.

2. Consider joining an active retired persons organization, i.e. AARP (American Association of Retired Persons, Washington, D.C.).

3. *Plan* for retirement early
   a. Living accommodations (is the present house too large or poorly designed for the aging person?; is the retirement home or village one that will impose adjustment problems or ease them?)
   b. Transportation (is public transportation available?)
   c. Long-term development of new hobbies which are not

physically demanding

d. Financial and health benefits (local, state, and federal)

4. Stay as physically and emotionally involved as you can. Growing old is as much psychological as physical.

5. Keep nutrition adequate even when it's easier (and cheaper) to ignore or skimp on essential nutrients and vitamins. Helpful information is probably available from the local county agricultural agent.

6. Consider retraining or even expanding community involvement. The little old lady with white hair can fight city hall if she is willing to try. Adult education is one of the most dynamic forces in education.

7. Contact with the following agencies can assist:

a. Local Community Action programs.

b. Easter Seal

c. Health and Rehabilitation Services

d. Community Mental Health Association

e. Social Security Office (this should be done well before projected retirement).

Chapter 8

MINIMAL BRAIN DAMAGE (MBD)
AND HYPERACTIVITY

THIS chapter is unlike others in the book in that two conditions are presented together. However, neither condition is necessarily related to the other, and a child diagnosed as having either condition may or may not have the other.

MBD AND HYPERACTIVITY

The two conditions are taken together for a number of reasons.
1. The labels are usually applied to children.
2. The underlying cause for both conditions is often said to be some kind of brain problem although the relationship is by no means clear and is rarely medically diagnosed.
3. The original reason for referral often is difficulty in school.
4. Both labels are overused, sometimes only to pigeon hole a puzzling child.

Minimal Brain Damage (MBD)

Unlike every other condition described in this book, the term MBD does *not* imply known structural damage to the tissue of the brain. Typically, the diagnosis itself is made on nonmedical grounds on the basis of psychological test scores and behavioral observations (usually on male children). Without a firm definition and a well-structured method of diagnosis, the diagnosis of MBD is often misused and can result more from adult frustration with the child than a clear medical or psychological condition.

The diagnosis of MBD is fundamentally based on a wide gap between ability (normal) and achievement (low) and may involve the following features:

73

1. Lowered learning in basic educational areas (especially reading) despite normal intelligence.

2. Minor neurological differences from usual children.

3. Distractability and impulsivity.

4. Motor clumsiness.

5. Other sources of difficulty ruled out as the cause of the educational problem including emotional disturbance, inadequate environmental factors, and medical or sensory abnormalities.

6. Visual perceptual or visual motor areas may be lowered below expected level.

This is not to say that MBD is applied in cases where there is a clear sensory deficit, i.e. the child whose vision or hearing is below acceptable limits. Rather, a sensory-perceptual problem exists at the level of the translation of the sensory input (i.e. sound, light) into the meaningful word or picture at the level of the brain. The child may see perfectly well and be unable to discriminate individual letters or reverse them in reading, i.e. "was" for "saw."

Even rigidly applied, such a definition works by exclusion, by ruling out causes rather than by discovering an underlying condition. Before accepting such a diagnosis, the parent should have contact with the following disciplines:

1. A psychologist for testing, at least including an individually administered intelligence test.

2. A physician to rule out medical causes.

3. A reading specialist (if reading is involved) either in the school or an outside agency.

The diagnosis of MBD should not be given or accepted lightly because of the emotional connotations associated with it. The label, as vague as it is, seems to communicate some vast and serious information. Any other favorable attribute of a child can be wiped out by the implied message that "he cannot learn" (overstated), and "he is brain damaged" (not found on medical grounds). Some words such as brain damage, MBD, and crazy seem to carry so much of an emotional aura that they seem to paralyze the higher reasoning centers of the person hearing it. Upon hearing the words *minimal brain damage,* the listeners hear nothing else and start behaving in a way that means "This child cannot learn but there is a good reason for it," which gives everyone (parent, teachers, psychologist) an excuse for not dealing with the learning problem.

What To Do As A Parent

Assuming that the diagnosis of MBD is firm, what are the logical steps that can be taken?

1. There is no single educational procedure or technique that is treatment of choice in cases of MBD. There are many reasonable methods that involve two major aspects:

(a) Good teaching methods that might be applied in many cases not labeled as MBD.

(b) More individualized educational prescriptive work for this particular child. The variability of abilities for child is even higher than is usual in young children and must be worked with. Learning disability classes may be available in the school.

2. The channels of communication between school and parents are vital to the educational progress of this child. The parent, without allowing his natural anxiety and frustration to antagonize the school personnel, should work closely with them in laying out reasonable educational plans and keeping attuned to any problems that may be beginning. In cases of MBD when the child is intelligent but is failing in school despite his best efforts, behavior problems can be generated by the resultant frustration and anger.

3. Consider the use of supplemental assistance and agencies for the child including:

(a) Tutors

(b) Reading assistance

(c) Learning disability specialists to work with the school personnel and with you

(d) Special services within the school including remedial reading, guidance, school psychology, and learning disability.

Sources of information about the above services may come from:

(a) The school itself — your first point of contact.

(b) College or university departments of psychology, reading, special education, and guidance.

(c) General community agencies such as child guidance clinic or reading centers.

(d) General or specific referral sources in your community including the "Yellow Pages."

(e) The specialty areas contacted in making the original diagnosis.

(f) The National Learning Disabilities Foundation or its local affiliate.

4. Remember that the key issue in MBD or learning disability is a discrepancy between measured ability and school achievement in the absence of obvious personal, medical, or environmental factors. If a child displays some of the symptoms that may be associated with MBD, but is progressing normally in school, the MBD diagnosis seems superficial and can be harmful in terms of expectancies. Sometimes a clumsy child with good verbal abilities and normal school achievement will be referred for treatment because of an anxious parent or teacher. In the absence of special academic or medical problems, the child's primary difficulties can be:

(a) Pressures or expectancies toward excelling in organized team sports that he is ill equipped to play.

(b) Communication, subtle or open, that he has some horrible, irreversible condition.

As ego damaging as it may be, not every male can be Joe Namath or Bobby Riggs. The clumsy child whose social and academic progress is adequate can be encouraged when he displays interest or aptitude in some sport but to push the child into competitive athletics on the theory that everyone should be an athlete can be damaging emotionally and physically to the child. Noncompetitive, but physically demanding, sports like recreational swimming or hiking can be of physical benefit without the connotations of pressure and failure that team sports may engender.

Outlook

It is probably clear by now that the author feels negative toward the term MBD. In the worst sense it is a wastebasket term, overly inclusive and probably consisting of a wide variety of problems having in common only a lessened ability to learn in the ordinary classroom situation.

The parent has the unenviable responsibility of staying in the middle between the child, the school, the home, and the specialists. Usually no one else will. How well the child's problem is handled will to a large extent be dependent on many interrelated factors:

1. Coordination and maintenance of separate programs which may be at cross purposes and are often discontinued prematurely.
2. The child's individual pattern of abilities and emotional stability.
3. Keeping the child from developing such an overwhelming sense of frustration that he gives up and becomes a behavior problem.
4. The availability of special resources within the community. This is usually more a function of parental awareness and militancy than financing and location. Psychologists and physicians usually are not very good at working with public opinion and changing an educational framework. Parents are more motivated and speak out on the problem when it concerns their child.
5. Remembering that each case is different and that highly competent adults have on occasion been labeled MBD in their childhood.

Hyperactivity

There is good evidence from research and common sense that from birth on, people are different in general activity level. There are lively babies and quiet babies with most falling somewhere in between. Falling somewhere beyond the active, lively child in general activity level and distractibility is the hyperactive or hyperkinetic youngster. Hyperactivity could be defined as a general level of activity and/or distractability so great as to:

1. Be significantly beyond the level expected at the

developmental age of the child. (Most two-year-olds are distractable and in constant motion and are hard to control.)

2. Sufficient to significantly slow developmental learning and educational growth of the child.

3. Be nonselective. The child cannot turn off his hyperactivity depending on the demands of the situation.

Diagnosis

Popular magazines have helped to publicize this disease label which is being misapplied to normally active children. Hyperkinesis certainly is a recognizable and important condition, but it probably does not occur at nearly the rate of diagnosis or popular opinion. One nationally distributed magazine estimated that *40 percent* of California children were hyperactive. Such a rate reflects the overuse of the term *hyperactive,* not the number of children who really are hyperactive.

Children at certain ages are active, distractable, and hard to handle. These attributes go with the age. When the child is noticeably beyond the level of activity of his peers, and especially if the developmental tasks are not being met as fast as other children because of this activity, then an outsider (pediatrician or child psychologist or both) should be consulted for an evaluation.

Treatment

There are two major techniques that are typically considered alone or in combination in assisting hyperactive youngsters: drug prescriptions and behavior modification.

Drugs: The use of drugs are prescribed and monitored by your pediatrician is probably treatment of choice in hyperactivity. When drugs work, they work quickly and effectively, removing a considerable burden for the child and parents. Usually the drug effect desired is the lowering of general activity level and increasing attention span and may involve side effects such as loss of appetite, sleeplessness, or nervousness.

However, drug effects are extremely individual. When your

physician prescribes a given drug at a given dosage, he is using his best judgment at the time. If after the drug has reached effective levels (days or hours depending on the drug), the effect is not that desired or if side effects (which you should ask your physician to describe) occur, then recontact your physician for his advice. Do not discontinue or modify the dosage without talking to the physician. Your physician must be kept informed so he can help you. If the child is going to school, his activities there should also be monitored. The drugs typically used in controlling hyperactivity in youngsters have a completely opposite effect on adults. The reversal of effect noted with certain drugs when used with children is called the *paradoxical effect*. When a child does not respond in the expected way when taking the medication, the physician prescribing the drug should be contacted immediately. In addition, if the drug does work and the hoped for "turn around" of behavior occurs, *do not* discontinue the medication without medical advice. Hyperactivity can improve with increasing age, but this is a matter of years, not weeks.

Behavior Modification: In conjunction with drug treatment or by itself, behavior modification can often be of considerable benefit in helping the parents of the hyperactive child. Briefly, behavior modification involves the following steps:

1. Describing the problem in concrete terms and measuring how often it occurs.
2. Determining what is maintaining the behavior (what reward follows the behavior).
3. Changing the payoff to change the behavior.

    The task is more complex than the simple explanation above. Among other things it requires that the parents become actively involved in the treatment and that they become very consistent in their approach to the problem once a treatment procedure is elected.

If behavior modification does appear to be one alternative to be explored, the parent may find the following book helpful: Madsen and Madsen, *Parents/Children/Discipline: A Positive Approach,* Allyn and Bacon, 1972.

Assistance in setting up a program can be obtained from clinical or school psychologists in the public schools, in child guidance clinics, or private practice who specialize in behavior modification. Popular books and motion pictures to the contrary, behavior modification is not brain washing, does not treat the individual like a white rat, and does not always work.

A Final Note on Prognosis

Hyperactivity is one of the few conditions that we really may "grow out of." Sometimes hyperactivity gets better or disappears at puberty. For that reason it has been linked to the maturation of a previously immature nervous system.

However, if a child is truly hyperactive and consequently does not learn at a rate appropriate to his abilities, he still has problems whether the hyperactivity will disappear or not. By the time a child reaches thirteen or fourteen he may have gone through seven or eight grades of school without learning enough. He is so far behind and so noncompetitive in an educational sense that he can easily give up on school and become a behavior problem and/or a dropout. For that reason, once a firm diagnosis of hyperkinesis is made, something should be done about it. Medical advice is the place to start.

In illustration of the enormous complexity of the problems involved in a child with minimal brain damage and the interaction of personal, developmental, and behavioral effects a series of three cases are presented at ages five, twelve, and sixteen. The reader should note the effect of the age of the child, the specific deficits noted and the home circumstances on the ultimate recommendations and prognosis.

CASE STUDY I

Age: 5-5   Referral Source: Neurologist
This child was referred for an evaluation by a neurologist who had begun a neurological examination of her. He tentatively suspected the possibility of congenital brain damage. Subsequently, he requested a neuropsychological evaluation with particular focus on potential educational difficulties of her.

OBSERVATION OF BEHAVIOR: The child was neatly dressed and groomed for both of the testing sessions. She presented herself as a very talkative and friendly yoqngster who was eager to see the "doctor." Additionally, she showed a distinctive tendency of being impulsive in her actions. On numerous occasions she attempted to start tasks before the examiner could complete the instructions, despite continually being asked by him to wait until the instructions had been given. Partially because of her assertiveness, and, also because of her verbalness, she appeared to be somewhat brighter than is indicated by her scores on the WISC. She appeared, however, to make a maximum effort on all but one of the tests administered, and all of the results listed are considered to be a valid representation of her ability. The one exception was on the Tactual Performance Test, which required her to be blindfolded. She tolerated this for a short while and then insisted that the blindfold be removed. As indicated above, this test was discontinued, and no objective results are reported. Other than this blindfold difficulty and her impulsiveness, the child was cooperative and worked diligently throughout testing.

INTERPRETATION: The subject's full scale IQ of 88 places her at the high end of the dull-normal range of intellectual functioning. A more detailed analysis of her mental ability indicates that, as might be expected, her weakest areas were on subtests measuring spatial ability. That is, based on the WISC performance, she shows a definite deficit in being able to manipulate objects and parts of objects in space. On the other hand, she demonstrated close to an average amount of ability on conceptual tasks and tasks designed to assess her acquired knowledge in the areas of general information, arithmetic, and vocabulary. Based on these results, it appears that her educational development is approximately in line with an average level of performance.

The neuropsychological examination provided a further validation of her visual difficulties. There were consistent signs of difficulty in terms of the translation of visual inputs into motor activity. This indication of constructional dyspraxia is consistent through three tests. Most marked of these deviation indications was a distortion in her reproduction of a Greek cross. Despite three trials, she did not approximate the simple geometric design.

Though quite sure of the problem existing in this area, it is difficult to make a definitive statement about her future educational difficulties. There is remarkable sparing of her higher level functions; whatever damage is present certainly appears to be static in nature, and she does show most of the prerequisite behaviors necessary for reading and writing. For example, she knows the alphabet, can read some beginning level words, can write her name, and can write the alphabet.

Socially, the child is developing adequately. Indeed, she shows some behaviors that are advanced for a child of her age. She is a socially oriented child, and the expected social behaviors of her age level that she does not have were acknowledged by her father as being due to her not being allowed to do them. For example, the parents do not allow her to go about the neighborhood unattended by them, nor have they allowed her to cut with scissors. On the other hand, she is reported to initiate activities with playmates such as playing school, where the child invariably attempts to be the teacher; and she crosses her legs and pulls her skirt down when she sits in a chair.

SUMMARY AND RECOMMENDATIONS: This child is a five-year-old girl who is presently functioning at the upper end of the dull-normal range of intelligence. She shows clear indications of a constructional dyspraxia, yet there appears to be a remarkable sparing of her higher level functions. Consequently, it is difficult to predict the possibility of educational implications. If she does experience difficulties at school, it probably will be in the areas of reading and writing. However, she has made good progress in learning the initial prerequisite skills in translating visual inputs into motor activities.

Because of her present behaviors in this area, it is doubtful that she will experience any serious learning disability. The father provided this information verbally in a follow-up conference. It was suggested that there was no reason at this time to coordinate this information with the child's teachers. Rather, it was suggested that he and his wife be aware of the potential problem and keep it in mind, but not expect learning problems to develop.

Additionally, the father was informed that no further

neuropsychological evaluation was seen as necessary at this time. It was recommended, however, that she be re-evaluated when she reached ten years of age.

In case of the eventuality that the child should develop problems in reading or writing, it was suggested that her teacher then be informed of the parents' awareness that such a problem might develop. And, if she did show these signs of having difficulty, it was recommended that additional help should be provided for her either through special attention from her teacher, or, if this is not possible, from a school psychologist or special educator.

CASE STUDY II

Age: 12-30   Referral Source: Neurologist

PRESENTING PROBLEM: This client was referred by a neurologist for a complete neuropsychological examination to assess his present level of functioning. He has had a history of school difficulty which may be due to residuals of nonpurulent mumps meningitis contracted during the first year of life. Of primary concern is whether or not his school difficulties stem from impaired brain functioning. Secondly, what steps would be appropriate in dealing with his school situation.

OBSERVATIONS OF BEHAVIOR: The boy was surprisingly eager and alert throughout the two testing sessions. He cooperated well with the requests of this examiner and seemed to be doing his best on each of the tasks. During the testing sessions and the breaks he talked freely about his interest in his father's work, plans for the future, favorite games, and his family. His cooperative, helpful attitude made the testing proceed smoothly. It seems likely that the test results reflect accurately his levels of ability at this time.

INTERPRETATION OF TEST RESULTS: The overall picture obtained is of a lateralized, mild, left hemisphere cerebral deficit. WISC Verbal IQ was seventeen points less than his Performance IQ, which was in the normal range. The score for the Halstead-Category Test was slightly below normal along with the Preferred (Right) Hand score on the Tactual Performance Test, the latter suggesting a left hemisphere involvement. As outlined in an earlier section, scores on the

Speech Perception Test and the Seashore Rhythm Test were lower than normal. These low scores may be confounded by the influence of his impaired hearing. In addition, his low level reading ability may have contributed to his low score on the Speech Sounds Perception Test. Therefore, a central deficit cannot be ruled out.

On tasks permitting a right-left comparison on motor tasks, such as Strength of Grip and the Finger Oscillation Test, motor functioning is equal to or above normal levels. Tasks which involve functioning, along with problem-solving behavior, as on the Trail Making Tests and the TPT, show a different pattern. Using the preferred (right) hand, scores were typically below normal levels, but the nonpreferred hand (left) on the TPT yielded scores above the normal level. Clearly again, one sees relatively diminished left hemisphere functioning on tasks requiring problem solving behavior. The best reflection of this impairment are his low scores on the WISC in the subtests of Information, Arithmetic, and Vocabulary. The obtained scores reflect a significant deficit in Acquired Knowledge, the sort of material typically confronted in school.

To round out the picture, the Aphasia Screening Test revealed a mild central dysarthria with a suggestion of dysgraphia. He is still far from mastering the cursive method of writing, as opposed to ordinary block lettering. He also has reading difficulty in school. These observations may serve to further substantiate the finding of the Aphasia Screening Test. On the Sensory-Perceptual portion of that test gross discriminations were within normal limits. On portions of this test requiring finer sensory discriminations, Fingertip Number Writing and Tactile Form Recognition, there was a tendency to make more errors accompanied by longer response latencies with the right hand.

Bannatyne Analysis of the WISC corroborates the aforementioned verbal deficits with below average scores on Verbal-Conceptual Ability and Acquired Knowledge. Visual-Spatial and Sequencing Abilities are both within normal limits. This pattern is consistent with his present and past school difficulties but does imply normal levels of functioning for nonverbal tasks.

SUMMARY AND CONCLUSIONS: This subject was administered the Intermediate Reitan-Indiana Neuropsychological Battery to determine what residuals may be present from a serious illness during infancy. In terms of general intellectual functioning, his scores on the WISC fall in the normal range overall with a significantly lower Verbal Score compared to his Performance Score. From this and other tests, it appears that there is a significant left hemisphere deficit when compared with the right hemisphere, as reflected in below average scores on test of verbal, problem solving, and discrimination ability. Motor skills are apparently intact and normal, with normal visual-spatial and sequencing abilities.

RECOMMENDATIONS:
1. A reading evaluation at a clinic and appropriate remedial action.
2. Contact the school psychologist and guidance counselor at his school to arrange for:
   a. Monitoring and possibly influencing his classroom behavior toward peers and teachers to discover possible sources of frustration.
   b. Arranging in-school activities to aid in the remedial process, such as a resource room.
   c. Exploring possible vocational programs in the school which would utilize his average (normal) ability for nonverbal material and de-emphasize his left hemisphere deficits.
3. Discuss with the parents and school officials realistic expectations for this student in terms of school achievement and vocational planning.

CASE STUDY III

Male, 16, no suspected difficulties.

PRESENTING PROBLEM: This young male high school student was referred by his counselor to determine eligibility for services. He has had a severe problem in learning to write and has never mastered cursive; he prints everything. Presenting information on his data sheet indicates "he has been tested and tested for this (his writing problem)," but no particulars are given as to when tests were given or what kind.

PREVIOUS TESTING PERFORMED: No records available.

OBSERVATIONS OF BEHAVIOR: J. was two hours late for the

testing situation and apologized to the examiner, stating, "I thought it was tomorrow." Questions directed towards his health history, manual dexterity, etc. were answered directly by J., but he could not remember very much about his fall. His answers to all lines of questioning were direct and limited; he offered no additional comments nor did he volunteer any information. J. was very cooperative, almost passive, during testing. The only change in his behavior was during the Halstead Category Test. His performance was very poor, and the test is designed to give immediate feedback as to right or wrong answers. As soon as J. began making mistakes, he began talking to himself, muttering under his breath, hitting the arm of the chair with his fist, cursing under his breath. He appeared oblivious to the examiner, and though his outbursts were controlled and contained, it was the only time when the case apparently lost his composure.

INTERPRETATION: Although few errors were made (only one on Trails B) on the Trails tests, the amount of time is unusually long in consideration of his IQ scores. Sequencing difficulty was evidenced especially on Part B; twice it seemed apparent that he could not remember the learned format of the test, and this, of course, slowed him down.

Scores were consistently high on the verbal section of the WAIS. Performance IQ score was depressed primarily because of his poor performance on Block Design and Digit Symbol subtests. His score on the latter test was low due to slow performance rather than any errors.

Strength of grip and finger tapping are within normal limits, although there appears to be a reversal of hand dominance on the scores. J. states that he often switches hands for various activities and sports, but indicates he was primarily right-handed.

Tactual Performance Test scores were slow, in view of his intellectual abilities. There did not appear to be learning present, in view of the longer time it took the left hand to accomplish the same task which had been previously learned.

Scores on the Seashore Rhythm and Speech Perception Tests are also within normal limits.

Acalculia and dysgraphia evidences appeared on the Aphasia Screening test, with an extremely poor performance on the Fingertip Number Writing, primarily with the right hand. On the test for astereognosis, only one coin was identified correctly by the left hand, none by the right. When the same coins were placed simultaneously in both hands, none were identified correctly in the right, all were correct when using the left hand. Drawings of shapes were "soft," in particular those of the cross and the key.

SUMMARY COMMENTS: Learning tasks involving spatial and abstract concepts are poorly performed. This showed up to a great extent by J.'s performance on the Category Test, where half the items were missed. The pattern of error on the subtests indicated that J. made fewer errors on the last four (of 6) tests, but learning of the concepts was extremely slow and total error rate continued to be high.

Slowness in performance on spatial items is substantiated by WAIS performance scores and slowness on the Tactual Performance Test. Cerebral dysfunction appears to be primarily in the right parietal area, with some involvement of the left parietal lobe. J.'s inability to learn writing would appear to indicate this minimal damage is of long standing and is diffuse in these cerebral areas.

RECOMMENDATIONS:

1. Examination by a neurologist. At this time the record of his previous fall might be obtained, since J. was living in Florida at the time.

2. For Vocational Rehabilitation:

a. J. appears to have a severe adaptive functioning loss to the extent that it presents an inability to make use of his good IQ and is evidenced by the writing problem.

b. Vocational goals should consider the fact that his tasks should not involve placement where use of his hands is of primary importance. The number of variables he must learn should be strictly controlled and limited in number. The task should not necessitate recognition of spatial concept skills.

SUMMARY OF HYPERACTIVITY RECOMMENDATIONS

Hyperactivity is often misdiagnosed and should show the following characteristics:

1. Higher activity than other children of the same age.

2. Definite problems (educational or social) in development

because of the condition.

3. Consistent inability to "turn off" the hyperactivity even if the situation is pleasureable, e.g. hyperactive children do not spend hours watching T.V., even cartoons.

Medical, educational, and psychological opinions should be sought regarding the condition but two treatments are often used:

1. Drugs (remember side effects and keeping the physician informed).

2. Behavior modification (absolutely dependent on a sustained effort and cooperation in school and home).

Chapter 9

EXAMPLES, RECOMMENDATIONS,
AND DEFINITIONS

THIS final chapter is divided into four major sections:

1. Examples of reports and recommendations relating to some of the major chapter titles.

2. General recommendations for any family who must deal with the problem of brain damage.

3. Definitions of any technical terms used in the book.

4. A list of helpful agencies and sources of information.

EXAMPLES

Stroke/Aphasia

This case involves a highly able individual who suffered a stroke while employed as technical supervisor. Recovery and prognosis are good but the expectancies of the individual have more to do with his degree of disability than the amount of brain damage.

Age: 40

OBSERVATION OF BEHAVIOR: This is a medium-sized, forty-year-old male who approached testing in a friendly and purposive manner. Except for the first meeting, he was on time for his appointments, and he seemed eager to begin testing. He was well-groomed and neatly dressed at the times of examination. At all times he was aware of the purpose for our meetings and he was appropriately oriented in all spheres. His attention was good and he was able to relate significant details of his past and present life situation.

Although he was generally affable and cooperative, he showed signs of fatigue quickly. He frequently became annoyed and frustrated with several of the test items. This behavior was particularly evident at times when he could not respond verbally. Several times he delayed testing progress by questioning the point (sense) of an item and by offering arguments against continuing. At these times efforts to elicit further performance were met with only partial success. Under pressure he became evasive, sullen, and irritable. Frequently he showed visible signs of frustration because of expressive difficulty. The general impression obtained from the interaction is that the man is acutely aware of the loss of skills, and that he easily becomes frustrated in not being able to match prior performance levels.

TEST RESULTS: The client is a forty-year-old referral from a nearby clinic. Although he appeared receptive to testing initially, later behavior indicated that this enthusiasm was reserved for items which were easy and familiar. He was sufficiently cooperative to complete the examination.

Tests of biological intelligence yielded an Impairment Index of .8, indicative of mild to moderate impairment of adaptive abilities dependent on organic brain function. This Index is in the brain damaged range but his performance was surprisingly good in view of the nature of his condition. The most apparent impairments were right hemiplegia and mild aphasia. These signs are consistent with a CVA involving primarily the left cerebral hemisphere. It should be noted, however, that the motor effects of the CVA are compounded by a prior history of polio.

The Category Score was in the brain damaged range but did not indicate more than mild impairment. This suggests that the patient will have difficulties in organizing complex problem situations and abstracting from them salient features which might provide clues to their solutions. The client is capable of functioning in a structured, minimally demanding environment however.

The Tactual Performance Test (TPT) Score also is in the brain damage range but again was better. Despite the fact that he was right-handed premorbidly, he showed good transfer of functions to his left hand. On the Hand Dynamometer Test, strength in the left hand was good. In two trials he reduced his performance time by more than 75 percent. This outcome indicates fairly good problem-solving abilities in a complex motor task. His performance on the Aphasia Screening Test reflected normal auditory and visual perception. Finger Agnosia, Fingertip Number Writing Test, and Tactile Form Recognitive Test results showed impairment in the ability to make fine tactile discrimination primarily to the right. The Trail-Making Tests were mildly impaired. He showed good recovery of learning abilities. The verbal portion of the Aphasia Screening Test showed minimal signs of dysnomia, dysgraphia, and mild discalculia.

The WAIS yielded psycometric intelligence scores which are also consistent with a CVA involving the left cerebral hemisphere. Verbal IQ, Performance IQ, and Full-scale IQ were 63, 106, and 81, respectively. In view of this patient's attained academic and occupational levels, these results suggest a minimum loss of thirty IQ points, primarily in verbal facility. Comparatively, the performance score is much better than verbal score, consistent with a highly lateralized lesion to the left cerebral hemisphere in recovery.

The test results generally show a deterioration of adaptive abilities but at a level much less severe than that which typically results from a CVA. This patient is able to approach a normal or near normal level of functioning on tasks involving attention, simple auditory discrimination, and simple motor skills. The pattern of test scores is consistent with moderate organic impairment of intellectual and mild to moderate impairment of adaptive abilities in recovery.

SUMMARY: The data are consistent in reflecting the effects of a stroke of more than six months' duration. Impairment appears to be strongly lateralized to the left cerebral hemisphere with mild to moderate impairment of higher level adaptive functioning, psychometrically measured intelligence, especially where verbal skills are concerned, complex motor activity, simple motor activity, and to some minimal extent, sensory and perceptual skills. In general, the test scores reflect remarkable sparing and would be indicative of fairly good rehabilitation potential. Since we are approximately one year past the time of the stroke, there is also the natural recovery function still ongoing.

Although the patient's recovery from such a serious illness is remarkably good, any decrease in his former abilities is totally unacceptable to him. For the client, his job was his life and he was remarkably successful at it. The man can no longer operate in the administrative capacity in the highly technical area of his training. Any lower level position is unacceptable and is denied value. Unless the patient can come to terms with his lowered, but still considerable, abilities, he will remain just that — *a patient*. It is strongly recommended that the total team expend every effort to help him and his family work through his denial and begin the admittedly painful process of readjustment. He is psychologically unsuited to retire and could still have a useful and productive life.

Closed Head Injury/Possible Seizures

This case probably represents one of the modal injuries for late adolescent males. Specifically, this young man was in a car accident. Although the original injury was severe, his age, general health, and good medical care have maximized his recovery.

DESCRIPTION OF SUBJECT: F. was a self-referral because of reported school-based difficulties following an accident last year. He reported learning difficulties, motor coordination problems, and some minimal speech dysfunction. He expressed concern about his academic future and seemed quite depressed.

TEST INTERPRETATION: On the Wechsler Adult Intelligence Scale, F. achieved verbal performance and Full-Scale IQ's of 101, 89, and 95, respectively, placing him in the average range of adult functioning. This is somewhat lower than the attained educational level and would call into question to some extent the right cerebral hemisphere, particularly when one considers the patient's past background as an exceptionally fine athlete. The split between verbal and performance weighted scores is insufficient, however, to postulate other than a static condition in a recovery picture. Examination of individual subtest scores was quite revealing. Arithmetic and digit span were both down significantly in relation to the other verbal skills. This might suggest immediate memory problems caused by the head trauma or could be merely an artifact of slight test-taking anxiety. In the performance subtests, digit symbol was significantly attenuated, a finding consistent with central nervous system dysfunction. In addition, picture arrangement was also signficantly lowered, calling into question in particular the right temporal area if backed up by other data.

In the tests of higher level problem-solving skills, test findings were unusually mixed, but in general indicated fine recovery of higher level problem-solving skills and adaptive functioning following severe head trauma but again tended to implicate the right cerebral hemisphere since there appeared to be obvious motoric slowdown on the left side. In addition and in support of other findings, there appeared to be some minimal signs of immediate memory difficulties. Again, it should be emphasized that considering the severity of the head trauma as indicated by the past medical records, the subject has made an exceptional recovery of functioning.

In support of the previously discussed findings which implicated the right temporal area, subject showed borderline performance in the speech perception subtest. Although lateralization is not possible in this particular subtest, it does call into question the temporal area in general unless the auditory mechanism itself is affected. On the Halstead-Wepman Aphasia Screening Test, the subject again showed minimal numerical and language difficulty. There appeared to be some very mild dysnomia and dyscalculia, but the findings are equivocal, and in general the subject self-corrected his efforts. There appeared to be right-left confusion and a rather subtle speech difficulty which was apparent, but beyond the precision limitations of the screening instrument employed. The equivocal language and numberical findings would be consistent with the Counter-Coupe Effect of a severe closed head injury to the right in good recovery. In terms of right hemisphere functioning it appeared to be mild but definite constructional dyspraxia again consistent with a recovery picture. The sensory and perceptual testing indicated no difficulties or suppressions under single or bilateral simultaneous tactile, auditory, or visual stimulation. Visual fields appeared to be normal, but the subject reported double images to the left. On crude confrontation, however, there appeared to be no signs of a gross visual field cut. Finger agnosia subtest was in normal limits for both sides of the body, and the more complex and sensitive Fingertip Number Writing subtest was also within normal limits.

Parenthetically, it should be noted that throughout the testing the subject experienced extreme difficulty in digital control. His handwriting was slow and laborious, and it was obvious that he did not retain his pretrauma motoric control.

The MMPI was disturbing in describing the patient's response to his present limitations. Patient appears to be quite depressed and to be withdrawing within himself in response to his own perceived shortcomings and to the real or imagined sights of the outside world. On the basis of the total evaluation of the MMPI without reference to the particular subtest elevations, it is strongly recommended that F. be offered psychotherapy and allowed to ventilate his feelings of inadequacy and hostility.

SUMMARY AND RECOMMENDATIONS: The picture appears to be that of a severe closed head injury to the right showing exceptional recovery of higher level adaptive skills but retaining residuals, particularly in the motor areas. It is recommended that F. be seen by a physical therapist and by an occupational therapist for evaluation of his physical limitations and for possible treatment. In addition, the minimal language dysfunctions found are probably amenable to speech therapy. The patient's borderline intelligence for college competition makes it imperative that he be made as efficient as possible in his learning skills. His reported visual difficulty may cause problems in reading, and a reading evaluation and treatment program may also be indicated.

Learning Disability

This final case is a fascinating one. We have here an adolescent of good intelligence who cannot read, and in consequence, is a behavior problem and was placed in a class for the educable mentally retarded. Included is a follow-up report after educational programming had been initiated.

BEHAVIORAL OBSERVATIONS: R. is a handsome looking male with no particular distinguishing characteristics. He came quietly to the testing session, reluctantly shook hands, and remained noticeably untalkative throughout both the morning and afternoon sessions. R. spoke only when spoken to and when asked for a direct answer. He listened carefully to what was being said and was very quick in catching on to what was being asked of him. When performing on a concept identification task, R. appeared to be very alert to the various aspects of the task although, in several instances, he was slow to discover the correct solution. In speaking to the examiner, R. frequently imposed long delays before his reply was forthcoming. When he did speak, his voice was barely audible, and this frequently resulted in the examiner's asking him to repeat his response. In those situations, R. would only reluctantly repeat his original response and several times appeared to give a different answer.

Not until the end of the testing did R. express an interest in why the tests were being performed and who was going to see the results. He also referred to several specific instances in the forenoon. At the time these incidents transpired, R. had appeared unconcerned. However, his questions indicated that not only had he been aware of what was going on around him, but that he was concerned as to what they had meant in relation to him. It is the examiner's opinion that R. is a great deal more perceptive of his surroundings than may be apparent on the surface. R.'s outward display of disinterest may be a learned reaction to frustrating situations and represent his method of coping with such situations.

Observation of R.'s reading behavior shortly before the time of testing indicated that for all practical purposes R. was functionally illiterate. He knew a few basic sight words, but phonic skills were practically nonexistent. His reading was also characterized by a large number of reversals and much of the time the words he read bore little resemblance to the printed page. He was able to match letters and sounds on an auditory basis, but was unable to make the transition to matching sounds with printed letters. His writing was also characterized by a large number of reversals, both of words and letters within words. Spelling was also markedly deficient.

DISCUSSION OF TEST RESULTS: R. was administered the Wechsler Intelligence Scale for Children in September. This test gives three IQ scores: a Verbal IQ, a Performance IQ, and a Full-Scale IQ. His full-scale IQ of 81 technically places him within the dull-normal range of intellectual functioning. However, this classification becomes relatively meaningless in view of the marked difference between Verbal and Performance IQ's. While his performance skills are in the low-average range, his verbal skills are definitely within the educably mentally retarded range.

R. was also administered a battery of neuropsychological tests sensitive to the integrity of the cerebral hemispheres. This battery of tests assesses a wide variety of abilities ranging from simple motor and sensory tasks to tests of higher level reasoning ability in problem-solving situations. An evaluation of these tests has clarified many of R.'s areas of strengths and weaknesses.

Reasoning Skills — Tests of higher order reasoning skills indicated that R. is, in many cases, slow to catch on to new concepts. In addition he has a tendency to perseverate on incorrect solutions and has difficulty in switching sets. R.'s reasoning skills which are directly dependent on language skills are particularly impaired.

Language Skills — Examination of results obtained on the Halstead-Wepman Aphasia Screening test indicate a marked impairment of language skills. This impairment is too severe to be accounted for either on the basis of cultural deprivation or on the basis of lowered school performance. Dyslexia, dyscalculia, mild dysgraphia, and marked signs of right-left confusion were evident. No difficulty was noted with the copying of geometic figures.

Psychomotor and Sensory Tasks Performance on the Tactual Performance Test was within the impaired range. This was primarily the result of poor performance with the right hand. Tests of Tactile and Auditory perception were error free. One suppression was noted in the right visual field under conditions of double simultaneous stimulation. On tests of finger agnosia, two errors were noted on the right hand, none on the left. On tests of Fingertip Number Writing, six errors were made on the left hand and three on the right.

Motor Skills Tests of pure motor speed indicated excellent performance with his right hand; although his performance with his left hand was slightly weak relative to his right. On a measure of strength of grip, he was mildly weak bilaterally with the left hand again being slightly weak relative to the right.

INTERPRETATION: Test results previously discussed indicate that functions dependent upon the integrity of the left hemisphere are markedly and consistently lowered. Language skills and left-right sequential abilities appear to be the most seriously impaired.

Although it may appear that R. is a "perceptually

handicapped" child, it is felt that his present reading difficulties are primarily a result of a severe deficit in left-right sequential abilities and not of a spatial-perceptual deficit. His perfect score on a recent Frostig test of visual perception and lack of distortion in drawing geometric figures confirms this notion.

Careful observation of reading behavior indicates that R. may be unable to match auditory and visual stimuli when reading because he may be hearing one sound-letter pair while seeing another. For example, one day in class, R. was being taught to read the word "stay." Auditorily he was able to recognize that the letters "st" made the sound "st" and the letters "ay" made the sound "a." When presented with the written word, however, his response was unintelligible. R. was then asked what the first two letters of the word were. R. replied "ay." When asked what the first letter of the word was, R. replied "y." Thus while the teacher was stating that the word began with an "st" sound, R. was seeing the letters "ay" because of his visual sequential difficulties. If one examines the nature of R.'s reading difficulties in this light, it is clear that remedial efforts must be directed toward improving left-right visual sequential abilities. These procedures should improve letter-sound matching skills and promote smooth word scanning ability.

RECOMMENDATIONS:

1. Despite the fact that R.'s full scale IQ does not technically place him within the educably mentally retarded range of intellectual functioning, it is strongly recommended that R.'s special education placement be continued for at least the remainder of this year. R.'s reading ability is so poor that to put him back into a regular classroom situation would result in more harm than good. His deficiencies in verbal reasoning skills, language development, and overall low academic performance make it imperative that academic work be structured at a level compatible with his ability level.

Considering the severity of R.'s academic handicap, it is slightly surprising that R.'s attitude toward school is as good as it is. Should R. be placed in an academically frustrating situation, such as being returned to the regular classroom, it is extremely likely that behavioral problems such as acting out or withdrawing from the academic situation would occur. Furthermore, since new remedial reading suggestions have been implemented in the classroom, R. is beginning to show improvement in these skills for the first time. To remove him from such a program at this time is definitely not advisable.

2. Should a learning disabilities unit be available next year, it is recommended that R. be placed in such a unit. If this unit is not available, his special education placement should be continued until his reading level is adequate for return to the regular classroom.

3. R. should be referred to Vocational Rehabilitation for further counseling and vocational planning as soon as eligibility permits.

4. R. should also be referred for a medical examination in order to more fully investigate the question of neurological involvement.

REMEDIAL READING SUGGESTIONS: These have been implemented at the time of this report.

1. R. should be switched to the cursive writing method with primary emphasis placed on forming the letters with a smooth left-right motion. Letters formed from right to left should not be considered as correct responses.

2. R.'s reading materials should be altered so that a line is placed down the left side of the page in a brightly colored highlighter. The first letter of each word should also be highlighted in the same color with R.'s being instructed to begin each word with the highlighted letter. Gradually, the amount of highlighting can be reduced until R. is able to begin at the left-hand side of each word without these additional cues.

3. It is recommended that R.'s sight word lists be separated so that only one member of any reversed pair of letters (i.e. "b" or "d") occurs on each list. Once R. consistently learns to respond correctly to one member of a reversed pair, the list with the other members may be introduced. In order to insure a firm development of left-right sequential habits, it is imperative that any one list be learned to a consistent 100 percent criteria before a new list is introduced.

PURDUE PERCEPTUAL MOTOR SURVEY:

1. *Balance and Posture*: No problems.

2. *Body Image and Differentiation*: There was extreme difficulty in imitation of movement; hesitations and unsureness were prevalent along with an oscillation from direct to mirrored imitation. Errors were recognized only after some delay.

3. *Perceptual-Motor Match*: For producing double circles using both hands, a characteristic "flat spot" was drawn on the lower inside area of both circles. During rhythmic writing, R. constantly wanted to position himself entirely to the left of the area within which the model was drawn and the imitation was to be drawn. During reproduction across the midline the left half was fairly inaccurate but some of the figures deteriorated even more after crossing the midline to the right side. Notably, vertical discrimination was lacking.

4. *Ocular Control:* Overall control was somewhat lacking, but more so with the left eye, especially in the vertical plane.

5. *Form Perception*: Organization was adequate, but the forms were not too accurate, especially on diamond-shaped figures.

BEHAVIORAL OBSERVATIONS: R. was noninteractive, nonverbal, and seemed somewhat shy, suspicious, and negative during initial periods of testing. These problems were overcome, to a limited extent, only with great difficulty. R. cooperated fully, however, especially in later testing. He actually seemed to enjoy most of the Purdue tasks.

His (overt) expressive abilities are very limited, and intermodal transfers (e.g. audiovisual, tactual-auditory) in general seemed below normal. At times, he seemed not to understand situations presented to him, but occasionally showed signs of high perceptual abilities.

This would indicate that R. has specific problems but is definitely not mentally deficient.

ANALYSIS OF RESULTS: The previous evaluation of March 10, 1973, is excellent. Of particular value are the recommendations made in this report, and further mention of it will be made later.

A subsequent consultation was held with his doctor in light of additional testing on the Purdue and Frostig surveys. It was deduced that R.'s visual-spatial and sequencing problems are subsumed under a genral problem of directionality and spatial relationships. Midline problems are evidenced in both the horizontal and vertical planes. Pure motor coordination is completely adequate, but perceptual-motor tasks, especially within and (transferring) across the midline area, are greatly impaired. This is evidenced by the low position in space and spatial relations on the Frostig and the various results reported for the Reitan Battery and the Purdue.

It is felt that, because of this general problem, specific reading skills were not learned which are realistically within R.'s grasp.

SUMMARY AND RECOMMENDATIONS:

1. All of the recommendations forwarded by the previous report are excellent, and each should be followed as fully as possible.

2. Continued SLD and special reading placements are definitely recommended, as well as continuation of R.'s vocational training in welding. Furthermore, materials relating to his welding class should be used, as far as possible, during his SLD and special reading sessions.

Of special importance are the efforts to remediate his reading problems. The fact that in three months he gained two years in reading ability points to the fact that this is an area well worth pursuing. The recommendations forwarded by the previous evaluation are excellent and should definitely be followed as far as it is possible to do.

SLD training should definitely be centered around skills needed in arc-welding, such as motor and visual-motor types of activities. Also, any other area that R. responds to should be pursued secondarily, especially those related to basic reading skills, using a multisensory approach at all times.

GENERAL RECOMMENDATIONS

The following recommendations are those broad enough to be applicable in most cases involving CNS involvement.

1. Follow the recommendations of your physician to the letter and keep him informed of any changes in the patient's behavior. Do not change medication without his advice.

2. Try to work with the therapists and become actively involved in the patient's total treatment program.

3. Stay with recommended treatments even if the patient regards them as punishing or childish.

4. The first six months of any recovery are critical. Seek the advice of your physician on any treatment (i.e. speech or physical therapy) that he recommends.

5. Consider seeking financial assistance with the help of a

social agency. Extended medical treatment is expensive.

6. The attitude of the patient's family is the single most important aspect of his eventual rehabilitation, but the strains of chronic illness are enormous. There will be times when you will feel very angry at the patient and guilty for doing so. If family pressures become explosive, seek help at social agency for counseling before the explosion occurs.

7. Definitely do contact the relevant national agency for information and assistance. A list follows at the end of the chapter.

8. Remember that many recoveries take two years even with intensive treatment and that damage to the brain, serious as it is, does not unquestionably destroy the patient's life.

9. Ask questions of those working with the patient if you do not understand a procedure or term.

DEFINITIONS

The following terms are used throughout the book.

Adaptive functioning: The ability to problem solve, to produce new solutions from available information, to think rapidly and flexibly "on your feet." In contrast to problem solving by remembering old solutions or old learned material. May involve language, abstract reasoning or performance skills.

Aphasia: A language or speech deficit resulting from damage to the brain, usually the left side of the brain. May be broken down into expressive or receptive aphasia depending upon whether the individual has difficulty in expressing or understanding written or spoken language.

CP: Motor deficiency resulting from damage to the brain. Causes and other effects vary. Is nonprogressive.

EEG: A painless and safe neurological test for indicating the electrical activity of the brain. Often very useful in diagnosis of various neurological disorders particularly seizures. Usually employed by neurologists.

Hemisphere: One side of the brain. In most people the left hemisphere controls language and the right side of the body; the right hemisphere controls spacial skills and the left side of the body.

Hyperactivity: A level of activity and distractability much higher than that expected at the child's chronological age. Often disappears at puberty but educational deficits before that time can produce serious future implications. Often controlled by a physician through medication.

Learning disability: Typically refers to a child, usually male, who

1. Is of normal intelligence.
2. Has no major emotional disturbances.
3. Comes from a normal educational and home background.
4. Is unable to progress at a normal rate in one or more important educational areas — usually reading.
5. May be clumsy in gross motor movements.

Memory disturbance: Can result from any damage to the brain and often results from severe blows to the head area. May be permanent or may improve, depending on the age of the patient, the kind, location, and severity of the injury and the time since the accident. May effect immediate memory, the transition from immediate to long-term memory, or the recall process of material that has been stored.

Neurologist: A physician specializing in the diagnosis and treatment of abnormalities of the central nervous system, including the brain, spinal column, and nerves.

Psychologist: A professional trained in the description and prediction of behavior; although often associated strictly with testing (intelligence, personality, brain damage, school achievement), he may also employ treatment techniques including psychotherapy and behavior modification to improve the patient's adjustment within his environment.

Seizure: An abrupt electrical disturbance in the brain, usually controllable through medication. Observable effects may be subtle or extreme. Often produces characteristic motor and consciousness disturbances.

Social worker: A professional in family dynamics and in the relationship of the family to the large community. Typically expert in the utilization of available community resources and agencies to assist the patient and his family.

Speech therapist: A specialist in the diagnosis and treatment of language disorders of children and adults including:
1. aphasia
2. articulation difficulties
3. delayed language development
4. stuttering
5. voice disorders

Stroke: Cerebral Vascular Accident (CVA). A blockage or rupture of the vascular system of the brain — usually produces a characteristic paralysis on one side of the body; other symptoms depend on the hemisphere of the brain that is effected.

AGENCIES AND FOUNDATION OF ASSISTANCE

Neurological Handicaps

American Physical Therapy Association
1790 Broadway, New York, New York 10019

Epilepsy Foundation of America
111 W. 57th Street, New York, New York 10019

National Epilepsy League
203 N. Wabash Avenue, Chicago, Illinois 60601

National Easter Seal Society
2023 W. Ogden Avenue, Chicago, Illinois 60612

United Cerebral Palsy Association, Inc.
66 E. 34th Street, New York, New York 10016

Speech Problems

American Speech and Hearing Association

9030 Old Georgetown Road, Washington, D.C. 20014

National Association of Hearing and Speech Agencies
919 18th Street, N.W., Washington, D.C. 20006

INDEX